A Practical Guide to
Acute Care
Case Management

A Practical Guide to Acute Care Case Management

The Day to Day

"How To Be An Acute Care Case Manager"

Resource

Colleen M. Morley, DNP, RN, CCM,

CMAC, CMCN, ACM-RN

DEDICATION

This book is a work of love and is dedicated to an incredible group of people who support me unconditionally. The opportunity to give back to my beloved case management community is a gift that I will appreciate always.

» To my children Caitlyn, Connor, and Cristian, my eternal thanks goes to my 'C Team' who let me practice on them from my ADN program through my DNP. You are the main reason for everything I do and I am so proud of the phenomenal people you have become. Know that you can do anything you put your mind to accomplishing. You inspire me to be a better person every day.

» To my father, Richard Morley, who taught me that excellence is achievable and perseverance is the key. Thank you for being an excellent role model.

» To Jeff Crofoot, who literally taught me the foundations of case management and became my friend, mentor, and partner in crime. Thank you for the knowledge base, encouragement, and proof-reading skills.

» To Eric Bergman, one fateful phone call righted my world. Your faith in me is a treasured gift. I am honored to call you a friend.

» To Mary Jo Cronin, my friendship with you has been one of the greatest takeaways from my membership in CMSA. Thank you for your support throughout the years.

» To Nancy Skinner, once and always, my idol and now my friend. Thank you for being an inspiration and cheerleader.

» To Ellen Fink-Samnick for lighting the way. Without your examples and encouragement, this book would still be in my heart and not on paper.

» To Deanna Cooper Gillingham, from the moment we met at CMSA National Conference, I knew this was going to be a life-changing friendship. I haven't been wrong. Thank you for the mentorship!

This book is ultimately dedicated to the memory of my mother, Patricia Anne Tanner RN CCRN, who ended her battle with Parkinson's disease on November 12, 2020. In 1976, at 29 years old with three children, she graduated from nursing school. I was 10 years old at the time and was inspired to follow her career path into nursing. After 30 years of working as a critical care nurse, she spent the last three years of her career working in case management. It was a rare gift to be able to mentor her during her career transition.

Contents

Contents

Contents

Contents

FOREWORD

A Practical Guide for Acute Care Case Management is an excellent reference and guide for case managers entering the acute care practice setting. As a fellow acute care case manager, a case management professional association member, and leader among leaders, Dr. Colleen Morley's ability to translate personal career experiences into professional career lessons for others is impactful. Dr. Morley is a uniquely qualified case manager and credits the "lived experience" of working in a new case management setting as the motivation for writing this book. She has written from the perspective of a professional who wants to succeed in a different clinical area from other case management settings such as workers' compensation, health plans, insurance, disability management, telephonic care management, or academia.

Fifteen chapters highlight the case management process within the context of utilization review, internal and external care continuum, transition planning, communities of practice, ethics, compliance, denials management, coordination of care, advanced directives, and other special topics. These diverse topics are presented from the perspective of an individual case manager and provide insight into the myriad of responsibilities for leaders of an acute care case managers. The book outlines the practical aspects of acute care management in a way that provides a roadmap for directors, senior managers, and supervisors. Leaders can use this guide as a resource for orientation, training, or competency-based assessments.

In 1997, I had the good fortune of enrolling in the University of Arizona's inaugural Case Management track for a Master's of Science degree in the Adult Health Nursing program. I did not know it at the time, but the pursuit of this clinical track would become a defining milestone in the trajectory of my career as a nurse and Air Force officer. The program offered a diverse set of clinical experiences that illustrated the benefit of case management in community health, managed care, workers' compensation, insurance, disability, health plans, and acute care. I was excited about the impacts that clinical case management could have on the most severely injured or ill patients who needed significant support and resources to heal, recover, and restore function.

I spent the next two decades of my professional career as an Air Force officer and nurse leader intent on institutionalizing professional case management within the Department of Defense's Military Health System (MHS). With the help of committed leaders from the United States Army, Air Force, Navy, and TRICARE Support Contractors, I successfully implemented policies, standards, training, coding, and reimbursement, multimillion-dollar contracts, and specialized programs throughout the system within the United States and overseas.

In particular, specialized programs were game changers in acute care settings dispersed across the MHS. Programs evolved throughout clinics, regional hospitals, and medical centers around the world. They were comprised of clinical practice guidelines, case management algorithms, specified coding for wounded warrior care, disease-specific specialties, and integrated care management. New positions, career paths and personnel contracts were developed. Transitions of care procedures were standardized between the MHS and Veterans Administration (VA), that provided safe, uniform, quality handoffs between the two healthcare systems. For over 20 years, the MHS has embraced clinical case management and achieved better health outcomes for patients and families coping with acute care needs. The ability to develop a leadership track for case managers was one of the most successful outcomes of professionalizing clinical case management in the MHS. The MHS leadership ladder resulted in case managers serving in executive positions at hospitals, regional TRICARE centers, and the headquarters of every military department.

The content and information in *A Practical Guide for Acute Care Case Management* will provide the tools and inspiration for case managers to advance their careers in both leadership and clinical paths. This book fills a gap in an area of case management that can be complex and overwhelming. Yet, Dr. Morley has successfully developed a guide that clearly identifies the most important topics necessary for success as an acute care case manager.

As a 30-year career military officer and health care leader, I am honored to pen the foreword for this book. It is an excellent guide, advances the body of knowledge for professional case managers, and Dr. Morley delivers on the promise of practical application. This book will not be a "virtual background prop" on a shelf, but rather a dog-eared, sticky-noted, and highlighted guide used by case managers and supervisors in everyday practice!

Melanie A. Prince MSS MSN BSN RN NE-BC CCM FAAN
United States Air Force Colonel, retired

A MESSAGE FROM THE AUTHOR

This book is titled *A Practical Guide to Acute Care Case Management* because it was created with the intent to fill in the lack of structured and readily available training programs often encountered in case management.

As a case manager, I found that when I transitioned from managed care to acute care, there was very little training available except for the new employee orientation process and on the job training. Typically, there is little formal education and training available to learn the role of an acute care case manager.

While there have been a few case management training programs developed since then, there is not a single resource that accurately provides clear information or training regarding the role of an acute care case manager. With limited references and resources, it can be difficult for interested healthcare professionals to investigate joining the specialty of case management.

As a director of Case Management without a budget to purchase formal training programs, I gathered resources, workflows, policies, and procedures to guide onboarding for new employees. This system has been better than previously available training. While there is still room for improvement, this book is meant to be a compilation of that information.

The information within is designed to be easy to digest and provide guidance on the day-to-day issues that a professional case manager might encounter.

The intent is to:

- serve as education for the new acute care case manager
- provide information for healthcare professionals interested in entering the field of acute care case management
- act as a day-to-day reference guide for the acute care case manager or a "one stop desktop reference"

As previously mentioned, I have asked many industry experts to contribute articles. You will find them interspersed to enhance your learning and understand the concepts presented. Each section includes a title page with the concepts in the chapter listed, a chapter specific list of references and a resource list with links to informative articles written by industry experts to help you put the concepts discussed in the chapter into perspective. I hope you find this resource to be useful and welcome your feedback for future editions.

Best Wishes,

Colleen M. Morley DNP RN CCM CMAC CMCN ACM-RN
Contact: cmmorley@altrahealthcareconsulting.com

ACKNOWLEDGEMENTS

As Deanna Cooper Gillingham said in the acknowledgements page of her *CCM Certification Made Easy*, "a book covering as many topics as this one does is not the work of one person." This sentiment is true throughout this book as well.

I am honored to have the input and expertise of subject matter experts, culled from known industry leaders, CMSA members, and Facebook CCM Study Group participants. My goal was to gather best practices from across the continuum that specifically impact the acute care setting. My secondary goal was to provide a professional writing opportunity to those who have the knowledge, but may not have had an occasion to be published as of yet.

Each contributor is featured in the Contributor's Index in the Reference Section of this book. Please take the time to read about this phenomenal team. I am indebted to each and every one of you and appreciate the time you took out of your busy lives and schedules to humor my request to pick your brains.

Kathy Samas Allen RN CCM

Anne Albitre LMSW CCM

Cassandra Battle BSN RN CCM

Eric Bergman BS RN CCM

Dr. Meghan Bisping DPT PT

Janet Coulter MSN MS RN CCM

Jeff Crofoot MSN RN CMCN ACM-RN

Erin Cunningham BSN RN CCM

Teri Dreher RN iRNPA CCM BCPA

Ellen Fink-Samnick MSW ACSW LCSW CCM CCTP CMHIMP CRP DBH-C

Deanna Cooper Gillingham RN CCM

Wendy Jaffe MSN RN CCM

Jared 'Jay' Johnson MSW LMSW CCM

Aishling Dalton Kelly CADDCT CFRDT CMDCP

Anne Llewellyn RN-BC MS BHSA CCM CRRN

Mary Jo McHugh BSN RN ACM-RN

Peter Miska RT

Ericka Peterson MSW LCSW

Metoda Posega RN CMSRN

Tonya O'Neill MSN RN CCM

Nancy Skinner RN BC CCM CMCN ACM-RN

Mariana Turgeon MSN RN CCM BSCS

Juliet B. Ugarte Hopkins MD CHCQM-PHYADV FABQAURP

Charles White EdD MBA

Ellen Walker LCSW ACSW

Anna Rheka Winkowski MSN RN CCM ACM-RN

INTRODUCTION

Nancy Skinner RN BC CCM CMCN ACM-RN

Nurses in a case management role have varying levels of knowledge and expertise in the provision of professional practice as a case manager. Some nurses were "poofed" (placed or assigned) to a case management practice without any understanding of the role or function of a healthcare case manager. Others may have sought a case management role as an alternative to delivering bedside clinical care to patients. Some nurses have embraced the profession because the primary focus of case management is patient advocacy.

Whatever the reason for seeking or accepting a case management role, it is essential to realize the duties detailed within a specific job description may not accurately reflect the daily functions of a case management professional. The specific responsibilities of employment cannot supersede or replace the foundation of case management that is detailed within established Standards of Practice. Two unique but complimentary Standards of Practice have been researched, developed, and published by the primary professional organizations that represent a cross section of case management practitioners. Both the Case Management Society of America (CMSA) and the American Case Management Association (ACMA) have presented clear and specific guidelines and definitions for case management.

The Standards of Practice for Case Management from CMSA defines case management as a "collaborative process of assessment, planning, facilitation, care coordination, evaluation and advocacy for options and services to meet an individual's and family's comprehensive health needs through communication and available resources to promote patient safety, quality of care, and cost-effective outcomes."[1] It also states that case managers are "recognized experts and vital participants in the care coordination team who empower people to understand and access quality, safe, and efficient health care services" (Case Management Society of America (CMSA), 2016).

ACMA also offers a definition of case management within their Standards of Practice & Scope of Services which states that case management:

> …in health care delivery systems is a collaborative practice including patients, caregivers, nurses, social workers, physicians, payers, support staff, other practitioners and the community. The Case Management process facilitates communication and care coordination along a continuum through effective transitional care management. Recognizing the patient's right to self-determination, the significance of the social determinants of health and the complexities of care, the goals of Case Management include the achievement of optimal health, access to services, and appropriate utilization of resources (American Case Management Association (ACMA), 2020).

Although these two definitions are unique, they share a common focus on effective communication: care coordination across the continuum of care and appropriate utilization of resources and healthcare services. Additionally, each definition clearly states the goals of case management include the promotion of patient safety, access to healthcare services, and the advancement of optimal health outcomes.

A practice of healthcare case management as detailed within these standards is guided by specific and essential responsibilities that each case manager adopts and embraces throughout their practice. Established standards list the common functions a case manager performs:

- Utilizing a defined method of screening patients to identify individuals who would benefit from case management interventions.

- Performing a comprehensive patient centered assessment that considers health risks "identified during the screening process" (ACMA, 2020), focusing on the "medical, cognitive, behavioral, social and functional domains as pertinent to the practice setting" (CMSA, 2016).

- Maintaining consistent collaboration with the patient/family/caregivers and all members of the transdisciplinary team to "identify relevant care goals and interventions to manage the patient's care needs" (CMSA, 2016). This collaboration results in the development of a care coordination plan that is "clinically appropriate and focused on the patient's care needs and goals for care and treatment" and is reflective of "patient choice and available resources" (ACMA, 2020).

- Facilitating "the progression of care by advancing the care plan to achieve desired outcomes while proactively removing barriers that impede the progression of care" (ACMA, 2020).

- Implementing and arranging "services among community agencies, providers, patient/family/caregivers, and others involved in the plan of care" (ACMA, 2020).

- Monitoring "progress toward the goals of the plan." Based on a continuing and comprehensive assessment, revisions to the plan are developed to reflect identified changes in the client's "condition, lack of response to the case management interventions, change in the client's preferences, transitions across care settings and/or providers, and barriers to care and service" (CMSA, 2016).

- Evaluating the "extent to which the goals and target outcomes documented in the case management plan of care have been achieved" (CMSA, 2016).

- Advocating "on behalf of patient/family/caregivers for service access or creation, and for the protection of the patient's health, well-being safety and rights" (ACMA, 2020). A professional case manager also advocates for "policy changes to improve access to quality, safe, and cost-effective services" for our patients and the communities we serve (CMSA, 2016).

The elements of a professional practice of case management as detailed above provide only a brief representation of the case management roles, functions, and responsibilities detailed within available Standards of Practice. Each case management professional is accountable and responsible for performing a comprehensive review of the standards and a comprehensive understanding of the roles and responsibilities as a case manager.

References

American Case Management Association (2020). *Case management standards of practice & scope of services.* Little Rock, AR.

American Case Management Association (2018). *Transitions of care standards.*

Case Management Society of America. (2016). *Standards of practice for case management.* Little Rock, AR.

Resources

The Standards of Practice for Case Management as presented by the Case Management Society of America are available at https://cmsa.org/sop (date accessed: January 27, 2022)

The Standards of Practice & Scope of Services as presented by the American Case Management Association can be downloaded at https://www.acmaweb.org/section.aspx?mn=&sn=&wpg=&sid=22 (date accessed: April 1, 2021)

Chapter 1:

Underpinnings

DEFINITIONS

Definitions accessed from Centers for Medicare and Medicaid:

- **Skilled Nursing Facility (SNF)** – an SNF is an institution or a distinct part of an institution such as a skilled nursing home or rehabilitation center, which has a transfer agreement in effect with one or more participating hospitals.

- **Swing Bed (SB)** – a swing bed hospital is a hospital or critical access hospital (CAH) participating in Medicare that has CMS approval to provide post-hospital SNF care and meets certain requirements.

- **Inpatient Rehabilitation Facilities (IRF) / Inpatient Rehabilitation Units (IRU)** – IRFs are free standing rehabilitation hospitals and rehabilitation units in acute care hospitals. They provide an intensive rehabilitation program and patients who are admitted must be able to tolerate three hours of intense rehabilitation services per day.

- **Long Term Acute Care Hospital (LTACH)** – certified as acute care hospitals, but LTCHs focus on patients who, on average, stay more than 25 days. Many of the patients in LTCHs are transferred there from an intensive or critical care unit. LTCHs specialize in treating patients who may have more than one serious condition, but who may improve with time and care, and return home. LTCHs generally give services like respiratory therapy, head trauma treatment, and pain management.

- **Occupational Therapy (OT)** – a branch of rehabilitative health that enable people of all ages to live life to its fullest by helping them promote health, and prevent, or live better with injury, illness, or a disability.

- **Physical Therapy (PT)** – a branch of rehabilitative health that uses specifically designed exercises and equipment to help patients regain or improve their physical abilities.

- **Recreational Therapy (RT)** – a branch of rehabilitative health that aims to improve and enrich bio-psychosocial functioning through active therapy and/or meaningful therapeutic activities to maintain or improve functional independence.

- **Centers for Medicare and Medicaid Services (CMS)** – agency within the U.S. Department of Health and Human Services that administers the nation's major healthcare programs.

CONDITIONS OF PARTICIPATION

OVERVIEW

Centers for Medicare and Medicaid (CMS) issue their Conditions for Participation (CoPs) as a guiding structure for various healthcare organizations to provide services and ensuring safe high quality care. In 1966, Medicare was introduced and CoPs were added to the Federal Register to provide oversight for the care received by Medicare beneficiaries. The CoPs provide a foundation for healthcare organizations to develop their reimbursement programs and provide care to all qualified patients. The CoPs outline the minimal requirements of care. The provider may go above and beyond the CoPs, but never below the requirements, to continue participating within the federal programs.

CMS defines the CoPs as "Conditions of Participation (CoPs) and Conditions for Coverage (CfCs) that health care organizations must meet in order to begin and continue participating in the Medicare and Medicaid programs. These health and safety standards are the foundation for improving quality and protecting the health and safety of beneficiaries" (Centers for Medicare and Medicaid, 2020).

Therefore, it makes sense that this guide will use the CoPs as the foundation because federally administered programs represent the majority of the payers to acute care facilities. Most commercial payers and accrediting organizations utilize the CMS guidelines as the source of minimal care expectations.

The CoPs that will be primarily referenced in subsequent chapters fall under the categories of utilization review and discharge planning. Additional categories that crossover include patient rights, health information management, and quality management. CMS provides Interpretative Guidelines to illustrate the expectations of the healthcare organizations and provide additional guidance towards fulfillment of CoPs.

The following list of CoPs specifically impact case management and has been accessed from published Interpretative Guidelines that are available at https://www.cms.gov/Regulations-and-Guidance/Guidance/Transmittals/downloads/R37SOMA.pdf

Best Practice

The professional case manager should have a good working knowledge of the CoPs as the foundation of their practice. The CoPs provide structure and guidance to promote quality care to all patients. Referencing the Interpretive Guidelines will help to understand the goals of each section of this book.

UTILIZATION REVIEW

§482.30 Condition of Participation: Utilization Review. The hospital must have in effect a utilization review (UR) plan that provides for review of services furnished by the institution and by members of the medical staff to patients entitled to benefits under the Medicare and Medicaid programs.

> 489.20(e) requires a hospital to maintain an agreement with a QIO to review the admissions, quality, appropriateness, and diagnostic information related to inpatient services for Medicare patients, if there is a QIO with a contract with CMS in the area where the hospital is located.

DISCHARGE PLANNING

§482.43 Condition of Participation: Discharge Planning. The hospital must have in effect a discharge planning process that focuses on the patient goals and treatment preferences and includes the patient and his or her caregivers support person(s) in the discharge planning for post-discharge care. The discharge planning process and the discharge plan must be consistent with the patient's goals for care and his or her treatment preferences, ensure an effective transition of the patient from hospital to post-discharge care, and reduce the factors leading to a preventable hospital readmissions.

> §482.43(a) Standard: Discharge Planning Process (a) The hospital's discharge planning process must identify at an early stage of hospitalization those patients who are likely to suffer adverse health consequences upon discharge in the absence of adequate discharge planning and must provide a discharge planning evaluation for those patients so identified as well as for other patients upon the request of the patient, patient's representative, or patient's physician.

> §482.43(a)(1) Standard: Discharge Planning Evaluation (1) Any discharge planning evaluation must be made in a timely basis to ensure the appropriate arrangements for post-hospital care will be made before discharge and to avoid unnecessary delays in discharge.

> §482.43(a)(2) Standard: Discharge Planning Evaluation (2) A discharge planning evaluation must include an evaluation of a patient's likely need for appropriate post-hospital services,

including, but not limited to hospice care services, post-hospital extended care services, home health services, and non-health care services and community based care providers, and must also include a determination of the availability of the appropriate services as well as of the patient's access to those services

§482.43(a)(6) Standard: Discharge Planning Process (6) The hospital's discharge planning process must require regular re-evaluation of the patient's condition to identify changes that require modification of the discharge plan. The discharge plan must be updated, as needed, to reflect these changes.

§482.43(a)(7) Standard: Discharge Planning Process (7) The hospital must assess its discharge planning process on a regular basis. The assessment must include ongoing, periodic review of a representative sample of discharge plans, including those patients who were admitted within 30 days of a previous admission, to ensure the plans are responsive to the patient post-discharge needs.

§482.43(a)(8) Standard: Discharge Planning Process (8) The hospital must assist patients, their families, or the patient's representative in selecting a post-acute care provider by using and sharing data that includes, but not limited to, HHA, SNF, IRF, or LTCH data on quality measures and data on resource use on measures. The hospital must ensure the post-acute care data on quality measures and data on resource measures is relevant and applicable to the patient's goals and treatment preferences.

§482.43(b) Standard: Discharge Planning Evaluation (1) The hospital must provide a discharge planning evaluation to the patients identified in paragraph (a) of this section, and to other patients upon the patient's request, the request of a person acting on the patient's behalf, or the request of the physician. (3) The discharge planning evaluation must include an evaluation of the likelihood of a patient needing post-hospital services and of the availability of the services. (4) The discharge planning evaluation must include an evaluation of the likelihood of a patient's capacity for self-care or of the possibility of the patient being cared for in the environment from which he or she entered the hospital.

§482.43(b) Standard: Discharge Planning Evaluation (1) The hospital must provide a discharge planning evaluation to the patients identified in paragraph (a) of this section, and to other patients upon the patient's request, the request of a person acting on the patient's behalf, or the request of the physician. (3) The discharge planning evaluation must include an evaluation of the likelihood of a patient needing post-hospital services and of the availability of the services. (4) The discharge planning evaluation must include an evaluation of the likelihood of a patient's capacity for self-care or of the possibility of the patient being cared for in the environment from which he or she entered the hospital.

§482.43(b)(5) - The hospital personnel must complete the evaluation on a timely basis so that appropriate arrangements for post-hospital care are made before discharge, and to avoid unnecessary delays in discharge.

§482.43(b)(6) - The hospital … must discuss the results of the evaluation with the patient or individual acting on his or her behalf.

§482.43(b)(6) – [The hospital must] include the discharge planning evaluation in the patient's medical record for use in establishing an appropriate discharge plan….

§482.43(b) Standard: Discharge of the patient and the provision and transmission of the patient's necessary medical information. The hospital must discharge the patient , and also transfer or refer the patient where applicable, along with all necessary medical information pertaining to the patient's current course of illness and treatment, post-discharge goals of care, and treatment preferences, at the time of discharge, to the appropriate post-acute care service providers and suppliers, facilities, agencies, and other outpatient service providers and practitioners responsible for the patient's follow-up or ancillary care.

§482.43(c) Standard: Requirements related to post-acute care services. For those patients discharged to home and referred for HHA services, or for those patients transferred to a SNF for post-hospital extended care services, or transferred to an IRF or LTCH for specialized hospital services, the following requirements apply, in addition to those set out at paragraphs (a) and (b) of this section:

§482.43(c)(1) –The hospital must include the discharge planning a list of HHAs, SNFs, IRFs, or LTCHs that are available to the patient, that are participating in the Medicare program, and that serve the geographic area (as defined by the HHA) in which the patient resides, or in the case of a SNF, IRF, or LTCH, in the geographic area requested by the patient. HHAs must request to be listed by the hospital as available. (i) The list must only be presented to patients for whom home health care post hospital extended care services, SNF, IRF, or LTCH services are indicated and appropriate as determined by the discharge planning evaluation. (ii) For patients enrolled in managed care organizations, the hospital must make the patient aware of the need to verify with their managed care organization which practitioners, providers or certified suppliers are in the network of the patient's managed care organization, it must share this with the patient or the patient's representative. (iii) [The hospital must] document in the patient's medical record the list was presented to the patient or to the patient's representative…

§482.43(c)(2) The hospital, as part of the discharge planning process, must inform the patient or the patient's representative of their freedom to choose among participating Medicare providers and suppliers of the post-discharge services and must, when possible, respect the patient's or the patient's representative goals of care and treatment preferences, as well as other preferences they express. The hospital must not specify or otherwise limit the qualified providers or suppliers that are available to the patients.

§482.43(c)(3) The discharge plan must identify any HHA or SNF to which the patient is referred in which the hospital has a disclosable financial interest, as specified by the Secretary, and any HHA or SNF that has a disclosable financial interest in a hospital under Medicare. Financial interests that are disclosable under Medicare are determined in accordance with the provisions of part 420, subpart C, of this chapter.

§482.43(c) Standard: Discharge Plan (1) - A registered nurse, social worker, or other appropriately qualified personnel must develop, or supervise the development of, a discharge plan if the discharge planning evaluation indicates a need for a discharge plan.

§482.43(c)(2) In the absence of a finding by the hospital that a patient needs a discharge plan, the patient's physician may request a discharge plan. In such a case, the hospital must develop a discharge plan for the patient.

§482.43(c)(3) - The hospital must arrange for the initial implementation of the patient's discharge plan…. §482.43(c)(5) - As needed, the patient and family members or interested persons must be counseled to prepare them for post-hospital care.

§482.43(c)(4) - The hospital must reassess the patient's discharge plan if there are factors that may affect continuing care needs or the appropriateness of the discharge plan.

§482.43(c)(6) - The hospital must include in the discharge plan a list of HHAs or SNFs that are available to the patient, that are participating in the Medicare program, and that serve the geographic area (as defined by the HHA) in which the patient resides, or in the case of a SNF, in the geographic area requested by the patient. HHAs must request to be listed by the hospital as available. (i) - This list must only be presented to patients for whom home health care or posthospital extended care services are indicated and appropriate as determined by the discharge planning evaluation. (ii) - For patients enrolled in managed care organizations, the hospital must indicate the availability of home health and post-hospital extended care services through individuals and entities that have a contract with the managed care organizations. (iii) The hospital must document in the patient's medical record the list was presented to the patient or to the individual acting on the patient's behalf. §482.43(c)(7) The hospital, as part of the discharge planning process, must inform the patient or the patient's family of their freedom to choose among participating Medicare providers of post-hospital care services and must, when possible, respect patient and family preferences when they are expressed. The hospital must not specify or otherwise limit the qualified providers that are available to the patient. §482.43(c)(8) The discharge plan must identify any HHA or SNF to which the patient is referred in which the hospital has a disclosable financial interest, as specified by the Secretary, and any HHA or SNF that has a disclosable financial interest in a hospital under Medicare. Financial interests that are disclosable under Medicare are determined in accordance with the provisions of Part 420, Subpart C, of this chapter.

§482.43(d) Standard: Transfer or Referral The hospital must transfer or refer patients, along with necessary medical information, to appropriate facilities, agencies, or outpatient services, as needed, for follow-up or ancillary care.

§483.43(e) Standard: Reassessment The hospital must reassess its discharge planning process on an ongoing basis. The reassessment must include a review of discharge plans to ensure that they are responsive to discharge needs.

Patient Rights: §482.13(a)(1) A hospital must inform each patient, or when appropriate, the patient's representative (as allowed under State law), of the patient's rights, in advance of furnishing or discontinuing patient care whenever possible.

Quality Management: §482.21 Condition of Participation: Quality Assessment and Performance Improvement Program The hospital must develop, implement, and maintain an effective, ongoing, hospital-wide, data-driven quality assessment and performance improvement program. The hospital's governing body must ensure the program reflects the complexity of the hospital's organization and services; involves all hospital departments and services (including those services furnished under contract or arrangement); and focuses on indicators related to improved health outcomes and the prevention and reduction of medical errors. The hospital must maintain and demonstrate evidence of its QAPI program for review by CMS.

Health Information Management: §482.24(c) Standard: Content of Record. The medical record must contain information to justify admission and continued hospitalization, support the diagnosis, and describe the patient's progress and response to medications and services.

References

Centers for Medicare and Medicaid. (2020). State operations manual appendix a - Survey protocol, regulations and interpretive guidelines for hospitals. https://www.cms.gov/Regulations-and-Guidance/Guidance/Transmittals/downloads/R37SOMA.pdf

Resources

Medicare Interpretative Guidelines https://www.cms.gov/Regulations-and-Guidance/Guidance/Transmittals/downloads/R37SOMA.pdf

ETHICS IN CASE MANAGEMENT

I have asked two Social Work leaders to weigh in Ethical Considerations, specific to Acute Care Case Management. Ellen Fink-Samnick is often referred to as the profession of case management's "Ethical Compass," and Ellen Walker is the most knowledgeable social work manager I have had the honor of working with. Their contributions in the area of ethics in acute care case management cannot be underestimated.

ETHICAL CONSIDERATIONS

Ethical considerations are an essential component in the role of case manager. Ethics for case managers can be broken down into five big categories: autonomy, beneficence, fidelity, justice, and non-malfeasance (Commission for Case Management Certification (CCMC) Code of Professional Conduct, 2015).

The "BIG 5" Ethics Considerations

1. **Autonomy**: Patient holds the right and freedom to select and initiate his or her own treatment and course of action and taking control for his or her health. The professional case manager advocates for the patient by fostering the patient's independence and right of self-determination.

2. **Beneficence**: The obligation and duty to promote good, to further and support a patient's legitimate interests and decisions, and to actively prevent or remove harm. Through education, the professional case manager shares with the patient risks/benefit associated with the options in the case management care plan.

3. **Fidelity/Veracity**: The act of telling the truth. The patient always deserves the truth. This may put the professional case manager at odds with other members of the care team or patient's family. Advocating on behalf of the patient for honest and open dialogue, according to the patient's wishes is key here.

4. **Justice**: Maintaining what is right and fair and making decisions that are good for the patient. This addresses equity of services and care to be made available to all patients as well as maintenance of objectivity in care provision by the care team, including reduction of the impact of implicit/explicit biases.

5. **Nonmaleficence**: Refraining from doing harm to others emphasizing quality care outcomes. Under every discipline or professional licensure, the expectation is to "do no harm." The professional case manager is no different, taking the concept further into coordinating a care plan for the patient that reflects effective, efficient and high-quality patient-centered outcomes.

Why Are Ethics So Important?

Understanding the underlying values and principles of case management is important in resolving ethical dilemmas, such as end-of-life issues, consideration of experimental treatments, refusal of care, decisional capacity, and other issues that can occur. Our ethical decision-making process is based on the belief that case management is a means for improving client health, wellness, and autonomy through advocacy, communication, education, and identification of service resources and facilitation.

Patient advocacy is an important part of case management that promotes beneficence, justice, and autonomy for clients. Case management advocacy specifically aims to foster the client's independence through educating patients about their rights, healthcare and human services, resources, and benefits. The professional case manager facilitates appropriate and informed decision-making which includes considerations for the client's values, beliefs, and interests.

Ethical behavior should be easy, but that is not always the case. It requires strength and integrity to take action yourself or to enable others to act. The professional case manager also needs to understand that there are different styles of ethical expression and must be able to understand and support others in their individual expressions without compromising their own ethics.

Commission for Case Manager Certification (CCMC) Code of Conduct

What are the core principles underlying the Code?

Principle 1: always place the public interests above their own.

Principle 2: respect the rights and inherent dignity of all their clients.

Principle 3: always maintain objectivity in their relationships with clients.

Principle 4: act with integrity and fidelity with clients and others.

Principle 5: maintain their competency at a level that ensures their clients will receive the highest quality of service.

Commission for Case Management Certification   www.ccmc.org

Ethical Issues to Consider

Duty to Warn

For those in danger of harming themselves or others, "duty to warn" refers to the responsibility of a healthcare provider to inform third parties or authorities if a patient poses a threat to themselves or another identifiable individual. It is one of just a few instances where a healthcare provider can breach patient confidentiality. Not all states have a duty to warn legislative mandate applicable to all professions. As of 2021, only 22 states have mandated duty to warn statutes and 19 states and territories are referred to as "may warn" jurisdictions. The healthcare provider is permitted to issue warnings about serious threats, but they are not required to make the report. There are four states that do not have statutes requiring a duty to warn, but this requirement has been established through court case laws. Six states have not clarified duty or permission to warn through either statute or case law. Three states and territories have statutes or case laws that expressly limit the healthcare provider's ability to issue a warning of this type.

Mandated Reporter

Mandated reporters are professionals, who in the ordinary course of their work, have contact with children, disabled persons, senior citizens, and other identified vulnerable populations. Mandated reporters are required to report or cause a report to be made whenever financial, physical, sexual, or other types of abuse have been observed, suspected, when there is evidence of neglect, knowledge of an incident, or imminent risk of harm.

Examples of mandated reporters in healthcare include:

Physicians	Foster Parents
Psychiatrists/Psychologists	Licensed Cosmetologists
Surgeons	Substance Abuse Treatment Personnel
Residents	Domestic Violence Program Personnel
Medical Examiners	Crisis Line or Hotline Workers
Christian Science Practitioners	Recreational Program/Facility Personnel
Registered & Licensed Practical Nurses	Emergency Medical Technicians
Social Workers	Teachers/Daycare Providers
Hospital Administrators	Real Estate Agents
Social Service Administrators	Other personnel involved in the examination, care or treatment of patients

Source: Data adapted from Manual for Mandated Reporters (2020).

These professionals can be held liable by both civil and criminal legal systems for intentionally failing to make a report per federal, state and/or local abuse and neglect reporting statutes.

There is no civil or criminal liability as a result of making this type of report, even if subsequent investigation determines the allegations are unfounded. Civil damages or criminal prosecution can result if it is proven that a false report was made with malice.

Individuals not mandated to report are nevertheless encouraged to report suspected abuse and neglect. Those who do report are protected from civil and criminal liability; however, making a false report constitutes a misdemeanor.

Decision Making Capacity

The professional case manager recognizes the patent's decision-making ability is vital to providing excellent patient centered care. However, there may be situations where the patient may no longer be able to make their own decisions, which leads to the process of evaluating the patient's decision-making capacity.

> Medical decision-making capacity is the ability of a patient to understand the benefits and risks of, and the alternatives to, a proposed treatment or intervention (including no treatment). Capacity is the basis of informed consent. Patients have medical decision-making capacity if they can demonstrate understanding of the situation, appreciation of the consequences of their decision, and reasoning in their thought process, and if they can communicate their wishes. Capacity is assessed intuitively at every medical encounter and is usually readily apparent. However, a more formal capacity evaluation should be considered if there is reason to question a patient's decision-making abilities (Barstow, et al, 2018).

The process to determine decision-making capacity must be followed precisely per your facility's policy and procedure because this determination can have an enormous impact on the patient, their ability to give informed consent, and to make treatment decisions.

End-of-Life Care

During end-of-life care, ethical dilemmas may arise from situations such as communication breakdowns, potentially compromised patient autonomy, ineffective symptom management, non-beneficial care, and shared decision-making. The professional case manager may be involved in advocating for the patient, clarifying communication, obtaining advanced directive documents from the patient or their family. Advanced directive documents can include a living wills, power of attorney for healthcare decisions. If these documents are not available, case managers have direct conversations with the patient or family members to determine goals of care or surrogate decision makers when a surrogate has not been previously established.

Assisted Suicide

Assisted suicide (also known as "assisted dying") is not legal in all jurisdictions. The American Medical Association prohibits physician assisted suicide stating that it is "fundamentally incompatible with the physician's role as healer"(Barstow,et al, 2018). Individuals who seek physician assisted suicide must meet certain criteria, such as having a terminal illness, proof of sound mind (decisional capacity), and the voluntary and repeated expression of their wish to die. These patients must also have the ability to self-administer the medications to complete the act.

Access and Coverage

Patients have rights to receive appropriate care (right care, right setting, right time). Entities must disclose limitations, exclusions, and financial conflicts of interest. Clinicians should also disclose anything clinically relevant or conflicts of interest that may impact the patient.

Confidentiality

Confidentiality is defined as "the state of keeping or being kept secret or private" (Fink-Samnick, 2016). Case managers are bound by a moral obligation to keep patients' information private. In the age of the electronic health records, there are challenges to maintaining confidentiality. Within any entity, a large number of staff may be authorized to enter and read clinical and personal information about any patient in the facility. Computerized medical records increase the possibility of a breach of privacy. Similarly, the use of laptops, with their portability (easily removed, forgotten, or outright stolen) and the ability to connect to facility information networks creates high-risk scenarios for breaches of confidentiality.

Consider these scenarios:

1. A well-loved and respected physician sought care at the hospital where he practiced. After his discharge, the Health Information Management department noted that his medical records had been accessed by over 200 hospital employees not directly involved in his care. Most stated that they "were concerned about him and just wanted to know what was going on." Those 200 people were either terminated or suspended according to the facility's privacy policy.

2. In 2017, a laptop stolen from a healthcare worker's car in Rhode Island led to the disclosure of over 20,000 individuals' protected health information (PHI). The healthcare provider paid over $1 million in fines due to the breach in protocols and not having protective encryption on all of his devices with access to PHI.

HIPAA

In 1996, the Health Insurance Portability and Accountability Act of 1996 (HIPAA) was signed into federal law (Public Law 104-191).

The intent of HIPAA is to improve the efficiency and effectiveness of the health care system through the establishment of standards and requirements for the electronic transmission of certain health information by combating fraud, waste, and abuse, and by establishing security and privacy standards.

The HIPAA Privacy Rule, located within 45 CFR Part 160 and Subparts A and E of Part 164:

» Establishes national standards for protecting an individual patient's medical record and personal health information

» Applies to health plans, healthcare clearinghouses, and healthcare providers that conduct certain healthcare transactions electronically

» Establishes limits and conditions for the use and disclosure of medical record and personal health information without patient authorization

 • Affords patients with rights over their medical record and personal health information, including the right of examination, a right to a copy, and a right to request corrections

Fun Fact: HIPAA was never intended to prevent the transfer of information. It does however, safeguard patient's health information. The professional case manager protects the patient's information, maintaining confidentiality by adhering to "minimum necessary" (revealing as just enough information to provide care) standards when communicating with payers, post-acute care providers, and others for business related needs.

There are some exceptions to the confidentiality rules:
 • You have received authorization from the patient to divulge information
 • Complying with a court order
 • Reporting births or deaths

Confidentiality and Social Media

» Do not post or publish any content on social media sites that contains patient details or identifying information (including photographs and testimonials) without the patient's permission and written consent. The consent should explicitly state how the information will be used.

» Know your facility's policies and procedures regarding the photographic use of cellphones and other mobile technologies.

» If you have a question, have someone who is familiar with HIPAA and state privacy regulations review what you want to post to ensure information does not violate patient confidentiality.

» Know HIPAA and state privacy laws and the consequences of violating these regulations.

» Understand the technical limitations and terms and conditions of any social media sites that you plan to use. For example, information sent via messaging functions are most likely not encrypted, and the site might maintain the right to access any personal information (Fink-Samnick & Muller, 2013).

Best Practices

1. **Trust your gut.** If it doesn't feel right, it probably isn't.
2. **Find an Ethics mentor.** Ethics committees and risk management are great places to start.
3. **Keep up on the changes in the law: Federal, State and Local.** It is your responsibility to know and understand how these laws and changes affect you and your practice.

References

Barstow, C, Shahan, B & Roberts M. (2018). Evaluating medical decision-making capacity in practice. *Am Fam Physician 98*(1):40-46.

Children's Justice Task Force. (2020). Manual for Mandated Reporters. Illinois Department of Children and Family Services. September 2020.

Commission for Case Manager Certification (2015). The Code of Ethics and Professional Conduct for Case Managers, The Commission for Case Manager Certification, Mount Laurel, NJ.

Fink-Samnick, E. (2016). Case Management Ethics 2017: Where Should Your Ethical Compass Point? AAMCN Fall Conference, November 2016.

Fink-Samnick, E. & Muller, L. (2013). Ten steps to navigate ethical, legal challenges in case management.

Fink-Samnick, E. (2019). The essential guide to interprofessional ethics in healthcare case management.

Morley-Wines, C. (2012). Ethical decision making in case management. AAMCN Study prep course.

Treiger, T. and Fink-Samnick, E. (2015). COLLABORATE® for Professional Case Management: A University Competency-Based Paradigm, 1st Edition, Wolters Kluwer, Philadelphia, PA.

Resources

CCMC Code of Professional Conduct https://ccmcertification.org/about-ccmc/code-professional-conduct

ETHICAL VERSUS MORAL DILEMMAS

Ellen Fink-Samnick MSW ACSW LCSW CCM CCTP CMHIMP CRP DBH-C

Ethics is a universal construct experienced by all case managers, especially those who work within acute care settings. These moral principles or values frame why people behave and act as they do in terms of what is good and bad with moral duty and obligation (Merriam-Webster, 2020). By definition, ethical and moral dilemmas are intertwined in ethical situations. The realities of ethical dilemmas appear daily across hospitals and span a range of situations that directly involve case managers.

There are three main categories of ethical issues present for case management consideration, which appear in *Table 1.1 Ethics categories on page 18* (Fink-Samnick, 2019).

- Clinical ethics or bioethics
- Professional ethics
- Organizational ethics

Some ethical circumstances are in the domain of clinical or bioethics and focused on treatment and decision-making. Case managers are often tapped to participate in these situations, such as working to reconcile patient capacity or competence to make informed decisions about their care. Amid the coronavirus pandemic, these types of ethical events have intensified.

As organizations are forced to deal with massive volumes of critically ill patients and surge capacity, case managers and their treatment teams have encountered tough life-altering decisions around triaging patients. Rationing care and supplies has pushed many in the workforce to the edge of ethical despair.

Another category of ethical circumstances relates to the ethical behaviors of healthcare professionals and case managers in the context of workplace performance and related interactions. These situations fall under professional (also known as organizational) ethics and involve compliance with expected standards of behavior for a specific workforce. For case managers, the standards or tenets include the principles of autonomy, beneficence, fidelity, integrity, justice, and non-malfeasance.

A synergistic and complex relationship exists between bioethics and professional ethics. Consider the complicated scenario where a patient wants to pursue all the options to prolong their own life, but this decision is counter to physician's recommendation. Care is deemed to be futile and affirmed by the facility's ethics committee. In accordance with state laws and organizational policies, you are instructed to work with the family to affect the patient transfer to a practitioner and provider that share the patient's perspective. The patient and family trust the care at the hospital and refuse to leave or allow the transfer. They prefer to find another physician at the facility to care for the patient and threaten to go to the media with their fight. You understand the physician's and ethics committee's decisions, but also respect case management's ethical tenet of patient autonomy. In addition, you believe whole-heartedly in the primary role of a case manager to be the patient advocate. Situations such as these become a slippery slope for case management.

Term	Definition
Bioethics (Clinical Ethics)	Situations to explore the philosophical implications of biological research and its applications in medicine (e.g. allowance of experimental protocols or treatments by a facility, treatment planning for clients with questionable decision-making capacity)
Professional Ethics	Personal, professional, and corporate standards of behavior expected of professionals; often aligned with established principles, tenets, standards of practice for the requisite profession (e.g. autonomy, beneficence, veracity)
Organizational Ethics	Standards and principles by which organizations operate; often aligned with organizational culture, mission, vision (e.g. fidelity, leadership, excellence, compassion)

Table 1.1 Ethics categories
Adapted from Fink-Samnick, E. (2019). Table layout by author.

Imagine another situation where you are case managing a 17-year-old adolescent diagnosed with leukemia. The patient adamantly refuses the physician's recommendation to start chemotherapy given the favorable prognosis. The family supports the patient's decision and requests a discharge order. The physician tells you to report the situation as child neglect to Child Protective Services. Where does your ethical compass point in this situation? Is the ethical responsibility to the hospital, the patient, or your professional ethical code? It's possible that your professional values contradict your personal and moral beliefs, if not also the law.

The final category of ethics involves organizational culture and practices. Imagine that you work tirelessly to advance discharge planning arrangements for a patient unable to participate in the decision-making process. You have worked closely with the family to accept the patient's inability to be discharged directly home. All vested parties are in agreement, but the patient's daughter requests to be notified about the discharge process so she can meet the patient at the facility to help smooth transition. This seems like a reasonable request in light of the patient's sundowning symptoms related to Alzheimer's.

The hospitalist gets to the unit later than planned and completes the patient's discharge and transfer orders at 8:00 p.m. You are working until 9:00 p.m. and are relieved to have the order. However, the patient's daughter works during the night and is unable to be reached. You leave a message on her cell phone and are unable to speak with her directly. The feeling of pressure intensifies as you hear the voice of the hospital's Revenue Management Specialist in your head citing the facility's explicit mantra, "when patients are ready to be moved, we move them out, no exceptions." The language makes your ethical eyes roll each time you hear it.

Suddenly you stop and think, "how would I feel if my parent or family member were transferred without my input or permission?" Thoughts about your former colleague come to mind where discharge delays were among the reasons provided for her recent termination by the case management director. You feel utterly squeezed between your personal values, ethics, and organizational culture. Do you face potential unemployment to enforce patient rights?

Advocacy is viewed as the primary responsibility of case management professionals. Yet, case managers can feel that heeding that responsibility may be counter to employer's requests, such as organizational fiscal imperatives for length of stay, reduced readmissions, and return on investment. What happens when the ethical course of action goes against a case manager's individual values, or even moral perspectives? How do case managers reconcile these situations? There are various ways to discern the nuances involving these various ethical, if not also moral, constructs.

Practical Case Management Considerations and Guidance

Moral Distress

Moral distress is a concept that began in nursing and has particular relevance for case managers. Think of the chronic discomfort which emerges from the rigor of juggling clinical, organizational, and professional ethics, with personal values. A case manager's thought process involves weighing competing priorities. Despite knowing the right action to take, you feel compelled to travel an alternate path.

For example, say you are case managing Mrs. Magoo, a patient with Medicare Advantage, who was admitted to the hospital initially for the COVID-19. Mrs. Magoo is ultimately intubated, but eventually she is able to recover. While she survives her rigorous hospitalization and treatment course, she is unable to be extubated. The family has been cooperative, understanding the need to pursue a long-term acute care hospital (LTACH). An appropriate LTACH placement is found, though a glitch emerges: the preferred LTACH is no longer contracted with Mrs. Magoo's insurance company. You review the alternative option with the patient's family, which involves transfer to a different LTACH. That facility has had several well-publicized COVID-19 cases across staff and a history of violations filed with the local health department.

The family refuses to allow Mrs. Magoo's transfer and is furious. You contact the managed care organization (MCO) case manager to obtain out of network approval, which she agrees to do. However, the process will take one extra day. The physician has written the discharge order and refuses to rescind it. You strive to balance patient (and family) autonomy with prevailing organizational pressures to effect a timely discharge without incurring extra costs. Your manager is on the phone, urging you to move the patient, and your ethical gut is screaming to do the right thing.

It feels impossible to keep each ethical ball in the air without worrying one will drop at any moment. High levels of stress from the daily exposure to these difficult considerations will take their toll on even the most experienced case manager. Burnout and invasive occupational trauma are frequent outcomes under this type of routine stressful decision-making. Seeking appropriate guidance and support is as critical as using case management's established resources.

Established Resources of Accountability

Case management's Established Resources of Accountability incorporate the formal hierarchy of resources to guide each case manager's actions (Fink-Samnick, 2019). Members of the workforce are accountable to a number of formal resources from the licensure organization, professional standards of practice, and organizational policies. With a workforce that spans the interprofessional landscape, it can be confusing for case managers to know which resource is the primary source of accountability.

The formal established resources are comprised of a mix of recognized official guidelines and protocols that start with state licensure regulations and practice acts that descend to professional membership associations. Examples of such organizations include:

- Organizational accreditations: American Nurses Credentialing Center (ANCC) for Magnet status, National Committee for Quality Assurance (NCQA), Utilization Review Accreditation Commission (URAC)

- Individual credentialing entities such as ANCC for board certified registered nurses (RN-BC), Commission for Case Management Certification (CCMC), National Academy for Certified Care Managers (NACCM), National Board for Case Management (NBFCM: ACM)

- Professional malpractice provider

- Organizational policies and procedures

- Professional membership association standards of practice such as American Case Management Association (ACMA), Aging Life Care Association (ALCA), Case Management Society of America (CMSA), National Association of Social Workers (NASW)

It can easily feel overwhelming to juggle case management's ethical and moral constructs in addition to the everyday activities of the job. When you find yourself in need of more specific guidance, remember that state licensure boards and credentialing entities offer advisory opinions upon request for their requisite members. Your malpractice provider can also serve as a valuable source of information and can potentially provide validation for actions.

Conscience Rights Rules

The current COVID-19 pandemic has been the most challenging professional scenario to date for healthcare providers, and especially the case management workforce. Employers are working to bridge the challenges between the needs of patients and staff's refusal to care for certain patients based on personal choice. A number of federal executive orders and state initiatives have been implemented over the years and faced fierce scrutiny.

In 2019, a conscience rights rule was passed for healthcare workers and was implemented at the federal level. The rule would have expanded other previously approved protections to allow providers, practitioners, and other members of the workforce to refrain from care that conflicted with personal, moral, and potentially religious views. This conscience rule allowed medical providers to refuse to render care that conflicted with their religious or moral convictions, and decline to refer patients to another provider with no such objections. However, the rule was quickly voided by federal judges by the end of the year (Fink-Samnick, 2020).

The conscience rights rule sparked discussions that focused on how the rule would be implemented regarding organizational liability and patient safety concerns. Examples of potential patient neglect were posed by various segments of the healthcare and behavioral health industry. There was concern that healthcare providers could refuse to treat patients, whether medical or in a behavioral health crisis, based on personal preferences about a patient's physical presentation (e.g., race, ethnicity, religion, clothing, tattoos, or body piercings). The thought that any patient could potentially be denied care under these circumstances prompted rescinding the rule. Those wishing to view the language of the original rule (84 FR 23170) may do so on the Federal Registrar website (www. federalregister.gov).

It is unrealistic for case managers to agree with or like every patient and their support system. However, the professional mandates are clear to not abandon or reject patients. Case management standards and ethical codes speak to integrity and objectivity in practice (ACMA, 2020; CCMC, 2015), with a case manager's primary ethical obligation to patients (CMSA, 2016). Case managers should be aware of professional reprimands through state licensure board or case management credential for rejecting an assigned patient. As case managers are beholden to the requisite regulations, guidelines, and standards, they should be familiar those reflective of their credentials. Case Study 1.1 on page 22 provides an opportunity to consider the complex situation with alignment to relevant industry resources.

Case Study 1.1

Marina is the assigned case manager for Dante, an adult male who self-identifies as gay and is admitted with a diagnosis of stage 4 stomach cancer. Dante is married to Marcus, who is actively involved in his husband's care and discharge planning.

Marina is a nurse who was raised in a religious family and does not acknowledge same-sex marriage. She is also credentialed as an Accredited Case Manager (ACM) and Board-certified case manager (CCM).

Application of regulations, guidelines, and standards

ACMA (2020): Scope of services: Assessment, Plan of care
Standards of Practice: Accountability

CMSA (2016): Standards J: Legal, K: Ethics

CCMC (2015): Principle 3: Maintain objectivity, Principle 4: Maintain integrity and fidelity

The attending physician, Dr. Shane, requests that Marina schedule a family meeting with Dante and Marcus to review the patient's prognosis and ongoing treatment.

In a discussion with Dr. Shane, Marina expresses reluctance to engage in the meeting or its planning due to her views of same-sex marriage. Marina expresses discomfort to Dr. Shane about her ability to be objective regarding Dante and Marcus.

Dr. Shane contacts Jose, the Director of Case Management, about the situation.

Application of regulations, guidelines, and standards

ACMA: Scope of services: Care coordination
Standards of Practice: Advocacy, Collaboration, Resource Management

CMSA: Cultural competence

CCMC: Principle 2: Respect rights and inherent dignity
Standards: Section 1: The client advocate; Section 2: Professional responsibility; Section 6: Conflicts of interest

Jose reaches out to Marina about the situation and requests a meeting.

A discussion occurs between the two professionals regarding how Marina's views have potential to impact Dante's care, her case management functions, and discharge planning processes.

Jose acknowledges the personal views presented her by Marina. He also presents how rejection of Dante could be potentially viewed as patient abandonment, which is counter to professional regulations, standards, and ethical codes.

Jose encourages Marina to review the documents so the two can define action steps.

Application of regulations, guidelines, and standards

ACMA: Scope of services: Education
Standards of practice: Accountability, Certification, Professionalism

CMSA: Standard I: Qualifications for professional case managers, O: Professional responsibilities and stewardship

CCMC: Rule 5: A Board-certified case manager will not violate or breach the standards for professional conduct
Procedures for processing complaints

Marina reviews the regulations that underlie nursing licensure in her state. She identifies language that speaks to not abandoning or rejecting patients in need, which is reaffirmed by the Code of Ethics for Nurses (ANA, 2015).

Marina reviews and finds the appropriate language for her case management credentials, and requisite professional associations. She also contacts her credentials for advisory opinions. Marina is committed to her role and understands how she must balance professional boundaries to assure patients are cared for appropriately.

Jose and Marina agree to maintain a continuing dialogue about how Marina balances her personal views with patient populations to avoid further challenges.

Educational opportunities are also reviewed to promote Marina's competence in successfully mitigating any presenting challenges and avoid harm to patients or their families.

Application of regulations, guidelines, and standards

ACMA: Standards of practice: Accountability, Collaboration, Care Coordination, Advocacy, Resource Management

ANA: Provision 1: The nurse practices with compassion and respect for the inherent dignity, worth, and personal attributes of every person, without prejudice.

CMSA: Standards, K: Ethics, L: Advocacy, N: Resource Management and Stewardship, O: Professional Responsibilities and Scholarship

CCMC: Principle 7: Obey all laws and regulations
Standards: Case Manager/Client Relationships

References

American Case Management Association. (2020). *Case management standards of practice and scope of services.*

Business Dictionary (2020). Professional ethics, definition, retrieved from https://www.yourdictionary.com/business-ethics

Case Management Society of America. (2016). *Standard of practice for case management.*

Commission for Case Manager Certification. (2015). *Professional code of conduct.*

Fink-Samnick, E. (2019). Grounding ethical excellence, Chapter 1 in *The Essential Guide to Interprofessional Ethics in Healthcare Case Management*, HCPro.

Fink-Samnick, E. (2019). Chapter 2, Understanding established resources of guidance for healthcare case management, in *The Essential Guide to Interprofessional Ethics for Healthcare Case Management*, HCPro

Fink-Samnick, E. (2020). Chapter 9, Emerging issues in *End of life care for case management.* HCPro

Merriam-Webster (2020). Bio-Ethics, definition, retrieved from https://www.merriam-webster.com/dictionary/bioethics.

Merriam-Webster. (2020). Ethics, definition.

Resources

Federal Register www.federalregister.gov

ETHICS COMMITTEES, CONSULTATIONS, AND CASE MANAGEMENT

Ellen Walker MSW LCSW ACSW

The Emergence of Hospital Ethics Committees

In the 1960s though the mid 1980s, Hospital Ethics Committees (HECs) were rare in United States hospitals. It is only at the end of the 1980s and through the 1990s that HECs became the hospital presence as we know them to be today (Hajibabaee, Joolaee, Cheraghi, Salari, Rodney, 2016). They emerged from different medical dilemmas that spanned many years occurring in 1962, 1976, 1984, and the last in 1990.

In 1962, the need for HECs emerged with Belding Scribner's development of the reusable dialysis shunt. This invention increased the feasibility of obtaining dialysis but created a dilemma because there were a limited amount of dialysis machines. This ethical dilemma arose because it was unclear who should have access to the limited number of dialysis machines and how it should be decided. Scribner formed a committee of laymen and medical personnel to determine candidates based on both social and medical criteria. This committee became known as the "God Committee" because it was seen as judging candidates regarding their worthiness for treatment. It also brought the awareness of the issue that "although medical technology can provide treatment, medical science cannot solve the value laden problem of who receives it" (Aulisio, 2016).

Other cases emphasized this dilemma to the public. In 1976, there was the case of Karen Ann Quinlan, Doe regulations of 1984, and the Cruzan case in 1990. Public awareness regarding medical decisions surrounded the questions of not only could medical implementation occur, but should it occur? The Quinlan case questioned if life sustaining measures should be continued if there was a poor prognosis for recovery of consciousness and low likelihood of life without technology. The Doe Regulations of 1980 brought a similar question to light about the controversy of withholding or withdrawing life sustaining treatment to severely impaired newborns. It initiated a wave of establishing HECs in pediatric hospitals and then in medical hospitals across the country (Aulisio, 2016). The Cruzan case brought up questions about withdrawing treatment, in this case withdrawal of a feeding tube from an incompetent person, based on the patient's previous statements of treatment preference. All of these cases surround the same basic question of "who gets to decide what for whom?"

A vast number of HECs emerged in the 1980s and 1990s. The number of HECs increased from being in 1% of U.S. hospitals in 1983 to more than 90% in 2001. One reason for this emergence was the endorsement of HECs in 1984 by both the American Medical Association and the American Hospital Association (Hajibabaee et al., 2016). Today, the need for HECs in hospitals is also motivated by The Joint Commission (TJC) accreditation.

TJC states in the standards of Patient's Rights and Responsibilities (2019):

- The hospital respects the patient's right to participate in decisions about his or her care, treatment and services (TJC RI.01.02.01).
- The hospital respects the patient's cultural and personal values, beliefs and preferences (TJC RI.01.01.01)
- The hospital address decisions about care, treatment, and services received at the end of life (TJC RI.01.05.01)

All of these standards of care statements have a direct bearing on the need for HECs in our hospitals.

Hospital Ethics Committees, Their Tasks and Responsibilities

Today, HECs are similar to the committee founded by Scribner in 1962. They are composed of a multidisciplinary team consisting of physicians, nurses, chaplains, lawyers, risk management professionals, social workers, palliative care specialists, and members of the community (Hajibabaee et al., 2016). All of these members provide a different perspective of patient care, but also bring similar principles to the table. These are the bioethical principles to be held by the members of the HECs (Anderson-Shaw, 2013):

- Autonomy (The patient's right to self-determination for healthcare decision-making)
- Nonmaleficence (Do no harm)
- Beneficence (Actions that benefit others, promote good)
- Justice (Fair and equitable treatment)
- Fidelity (Being faithful to one's obligations)
- Veracity (Honesty)

These principles are needed for the HEC to fulfill their three major tasks in a hospital setting. First, to assist in creation of hospital policy. Second, to make recommendations on individual cases. Third, to serve as advisors and educators, rather than decisions makers (AMA Principles of Medical Ethics 10.7). For our purposes, we will limit our information to the recommendation on individual cases, more commonly known as an "ethics consult."

> An ethical consult can be called when an individual must make a decision about which choice is best. Second, there must be different courses of action to choose from and thirdly, no matter which course of action is chosen, some ethical principle will be compromised. In other words, there is no perfect solution (Allen, 2012).

Types of consults include end-of-life discussion, use of life sustaining measures, conflicting decisions between family members regarding patient care, non-beneficial care, and discrepancies between advanced directives and care provided. All of these are situations in which care planning can be affected and the case manager would be involved (Cesta, 2011).

Once a consult has been called, the HEC will review the situation. A commonly used analysis approach is the Four-Box method of Ethical Analysis by Johnson, Siegler and Winslade. The four-box method looks at four views of the situation: Medical Indications, Patient Preferences, Quality of Life, and Contextual Features.

Medical Indications: This looks at the principles of beneficence and nonmalfeasance. The discussion will include questions regarding the patient's medical condition, goals of treatment, and patient's prognosis.

Patient Preferences: This view includes the respect for autonomy. What does the patient want? If the patient has decision-making capacity, what does the patient believe about the conditions and course of treatment planned? Does the patient understand the pros and cons of treatment? If the patient is not decisional, what does the advanced directive (power of attorney) state? If no other opinions are available, what does the surrogate decision-maker state? What does the patient or representative choose?

Quality of life: Beneficences, nonmalfeasance, and the respect for autonomy are considered here. Questions raised are surround prognosis. What are the issues restraining the patient's quality of life? What are possible outcomes for the patient with or without treatment? What is the current care plan for the patient?

Contextual Factors: The focus is respect for autonomy, but also justice. The HEC can look at financial issues and circumstantial factors. What are the family pressures or values at play? What are the patient's spiritual beliefs? Educational, legal, and research issues are considered as well (Anderson-Shaw, 2013).

The HEC meets together. They may ask for input from the primary physician, the family, nurses, and specialists caring for the patient prior to determining the best course of action. Keep in mind, that this is a consult. It is not a decision of what is right or wrong, but determining what is the best decision that can be made based on the information that has been presented at the time. This decision is expected to be taken under advisement, not to be the determining factor of treatment.

Case Study 1.2 on page 28 depicts a typical ethical dilemma for case managers in hospital settings. Do we keep providing treatment that isn't providing improvement, but is keeping him alive because that is what a family member wants? Or should treatment be discontinued based on the available assessments that he has a very poor prognosis, treatment would continue to cause him pain and suffering, and the patient's own stated wishes documented by the provider? This decision is made more difficult because Mr. George did not have an advanced directive document addressing his end-of-life wishes.

Case Study 1.2

Mr. George is a 78-year-old male. He has a history of end-stage renal disease, a cardiac condition, and congestive heart failure, which has been worsening over the past year. Mr. George had a respiratory arrest at home, was brought to the hospital, and placed on a ventilator. He was showing minimal response to treatment and he was unconscious. Fluid was building up in his system and he needed medication to keep his blood pressure up. All available data and medical assessments showed a poor prognosis.

An ethics committee consult was called by a nurse who stated she felt the care was not beneficial. She thought the patient, whom she had known before, would not have wanted the continued treatment. There were no advanced directives available to make his wishes known.

The family did not know what the patient's wishes would have been, but one family member believed that everything should be done for him. The resident on the case had previously documented a conversation with the patient where the patient had stated that he did not want to be kept on a ventilator without hope of being successfully taken off.

Case Management and Ethics Consults

As one can see, everyday cases can be infused with ethical dilemmas. Case managers are in a unique position to be able to see the concerns from both the medical and social perspectives. Case managers hold the role of being a patient advocate by enabling self-determination (NASW, 2017 and CMSA, 2018). "Patient advocacy relates to the ethical principal of beneficence and they work to advance the best interest of the patient and the family" (Cesta, 2019).

Whether as a team member of the HEC or as a staff member in the hospital, case managers participate in ethical decision-making. We do this by informing patients and families of their options for care and doing our best to ensure that their choices are followed. Additionally, we initiate ethical consults when they are needed and put patients' and families' interests in the forefront (Cesta, 2012). In turn, ethical consults can assist case managers in ensuring that their patients' decisions are being followed and the consults can also prevent delays in treatment as decisions are made comprehensively.

Case managers need to be aware of ethical concerns in their own practice. It is essential to provide care options to allow the patient to make a choice. In addition, there is pressure from third-party payers that may conflict with what is best for patients. In some instances, the medical institution itself may be the source of conflict. For example, concern over reducing the length of stay versus the patient's needs that would prolong care and therefore increase the length of stay. It is these dilemmas that should be made known in ethical consults to assist the case manager and the HEC (Bankston, White, Birmingham, 2015).

Ethical consults are not only enriched by the input of case managers, but are also a source of assistance. Healthcare providers should be knowledgeable about the benefits of HECs because of their assistance in patient care. It is important for healthcare providers to be willing to request an ethical consult when needed. Their input is essential to providing best patient outcomes. Case managers are in unique position to be able to do both.

References

Anderson-Shaw, L. (2013). The ethics consult process. UIC Ethics Consult Service, Live presentation, June 25, 2013.

Ausilio, M. (2016). Why did hospital ethics committees emerge in the U.S.? *AMA Journal of Ethics, 18*(5), 546-553.

Case Management Society of America (2016). CMSA Standards of Practice.

Cesta, T. (2011). Every day, the case management department faces multiple dilemmas over ethics. *Case Management Insider, 19*(8), 118-9.

Hajibabaee, F., Joolaee, S., Cheraghi, M. A., Salari, P., & Rodney, P. (2016). Hospital/clinical ethics committees' notion: An overview. *Journal of Medical Ethics and History of Medicine*, 9, 17.

National Association of Social Workers. (2013). NASW Standards of Practice for Social Work Case Management.

Rosner F. (1985). Hospital medical ethics committees: A review of their development. *Journal of the American Medical Association, 253*(18), 2693–2697. doi:10.1001/jama.1985.03350420105027

The Joint Commission (2019). Patient Rights and Responsibilities.

Chapter 2:

Utilization Management

THE UTILIZATION MANAGEMENT PROCESS

Utilization Management Conditions of Participation

§482.30 Condition of Participation: Utilization Review. The hospital must have in effect a utilization review (UR) plan that provides for review of services furnished by the institution and by members of the medical staff to patients entitled to benefits under the Medicare and Medicaid programs.

UTILIZATION MANAGEMENT PLAN

"Utilization Management Plan" refers to the hospital-wide plan that contains the essential requirements for the establishment and implementation of a utilization management process. This plan details the quality, appropriateness, and efficiency of care and resources furnished by the hospital and medical staff. The purpose of the utilization management plan (UM Plan) is to ensure that all patients receive medically necessary and appropriate care at the appropriate time and in the appropriate setting.

Acute care facilities develop a UM Plan incorporating the definitions and procedures set forth in the Center for Medicare and Medicaid Conditions of Participation, to govern utilization management processes in their facilities. The facility may add to its UM Plan hospital-specific utilization management procedures required by the medical staff, its Utilization Management Committee (the "UM Committee" or "Committee"), or state regulatory agencies. The facility's UM Committee, the Medical Executive Committee, and the Governing Board must review and evaluate its UM Plan at least once a year to make revisions.

The purpose of the UM Plan is to:
- Assess and improve the delivery of quality care to all patients, regardless of payment source, in an efficient and cost-effective manner.
- Delineate the methods for conducting reviews of appropriateness and medical necessity of admission, appropriateness of setting (level of care), duration of stay, continued stay, day and cost outliers, supportive services, discharge planning, and professional services furnished including drugs and biologicals.
- Assist in the promotion and maintenance of high-quality care through analysis, review, and evaluation of clinical practices within the hospital.
- Assure continuity of patient care. Address over/under utilization and scheduling of resources.

- Ensure the appropriateness, clinical necessity, and timeliness of support services provided directly by the hospital, or by referral contracts through concurrent review.
- Act as an educational stimulus through the review of medical records and study of patient patterns.

The role of the professional case manager in relation to the UM Plan involves the function of UR. This process is accomplished by reviewing properly authenticated documentation in the medical record and applying the designated utilization review criteria objectively across the patient's length of stay. It is important for the case manager to be familiar with the facility's UM Plan to understand the expectations of their role and the process for the individual facility. The guidelines issued by CMS are the minimum requirement, but each facility may customize their UM Plan to exceed the published minimum requirements, creating differences between facilities.

STATUS MANAGEMENT

Hospital admission decisions are complex clinical judgments formulated by physicians after careful consideration of numerous factors including the severity of each patient's condition, the likelihood of adverse events, patient medical history, hospital bylaws, and hospital admission policies. Medicare policy recognizes the physician responsible for a patient's care at the hospital is also responsible for deciding whether that patient should be admitted as an inpatient. The objective of status management is to assist in the determination of the appropriateness of setting (level of care), through the duration of the patient's stay in the acute facility. A patient's status or level of care in the acute facility can be identified as inpatient, observation, outpatient in a bed, or extended recovery. Inpatient and outpatient statuses are the only two determinations recognized by Medicare.

Definitions

Inpatient: The decision for inpatient hospital admission is a complex medical decision based on a physician's judgment and the need for medically necessary hospital care. An inpatient admission is generally appropriate when the patient is expected to need two or more midnights of medically necessary hospital care. Historically, the physician must order such an admission and the hospital must formally admit the patient as inpatient.

The Final Rule regarding hospital admission under Medicare Part A (42 C.F.R. § 412.3) implemented on October 1, 2018, included a clause to remove the then current requirement that an inpatient admission order "must be present in the medical record and be supported by the physician admission and progress notes, in order for the hospital to be paid for hospital inpatient services under Medicare Part A." As a result, CMS "no longer required a written inpatient admission order to be present in the medical record as a specific condition of Medicare Part A payment (Duffy & Ferreone, 2018).

CMS adopted the change in the Final Rule in response to reports of claims for medically necessary admissions being denied as a result of "technical discrepancies with the documentation of inpatient admission orders," such as missing or late signatures (signed post-discharge).

> It took CMS more than four years to realize that their contractors were denying admissions solely because the admission order was not authenticated prior to discharge. Once they realized what was happening, they proposed and then formally removed the admission order as a condition of payment, a change that became effective on Oct. 1, 2018. In the 2019 IPPS Proposed Rule, CMS stated, "it was not our intent when we finalized the admission order documentation requirements that they should by themselves lead to the denial of payment for otherwise medically reasonable and necessary inpatient stays (Hirsch, 2018).

Outpatient levels of care: The patient is considered an outpatient if are receiving emergency department services, observation services, outpatient surgery, lab tests, imaging services, or any other hospital services where the physician hasn't written an order to formally admit the patient as an inpatient. In these cases, the patient remains as an outpatient even if they spend the night in the hospital.

Observation: When a physician orders that a patient be placed under observation, the patient's status is outpatient. The purpose of observation is to determine the need for further treatment or inpatient admission. A patient in observation may improve and be released or be admitted as an inpatient (Center for Medicare and Medicaid Medicare Benefit Policy Manual, Ch. 6, Section 20.6).

Observation care is described by the Medicare program as a well-defined set of clinically appropriate services that includes short term treatment, assessment, and reassessment before a decision can be made as to whether a patient can be discharged or requires further treatment as an inpatient. Observation care is not defined by time, such as 24-48 hours. There is a desire for determination on observation cases to either convert to inpatient status if further medical interventions are needed or to continue care outside of the facility as soon as is feasible.

Unofficial statuses: "Extended recovery" and "outpatient in a bed" are not Medicare terms. These terms were developed by hospitals to distinguish between certain outpatient areas or to classify patients for billing purposes (Zelem, 2018).

Extended recovery: While not an "official" Medicare status, extended recovery is addressed by Medicare. In cases where a patient may have a surgical procedure as an outpatient, their status may be extended recovery if they require more time to recover that does not meet the higher status level of care for observation. The Medicare Benefit Policy Manual, Chapter 1, Section 10 states:

> when patients with known diagnoses enter a hospital for a specific minor surgical procedure or other treatment that is expected to keep them in the hospital for only a few hours (i.e.,

less than 24 hours), they are considered outpatients for coverage purposes regardless of the hour they came to the hospital, whether they used a bed, and whether they remained in the hospital past midnight (Center for Medicare and Medicaid, 2017).

Outpatient in a bed: The outpatient in a bed unofficial status has been used to classify patients occupying acute care beds in a hospital without demonstrated medical necessity. This status can be used while awaiting transition planning from outpatient services. This could include a patient in the emergency department, a patient receiving IV infusions, or a patient on hemodialysis that has no other identified medical necessity for admission (Sallee, 2018).

References

Center for Medicare and Medicaid. (2017). Medicare Policy Manual.

Duffy, C. & Ferreone, A. (2018). CMS Revises Hospital Inpatient Admission Order Documentation Requirements. HealthLaw Diagnosis.

Hirsch, R. (2018). Inpatient Admission Order Regulations Continue to Confound. RAC Monitor. https://www.racmonitor.com/inpatient-admission-order-regulations-continue-to-confound

Sallee, L. (2018). Patient status: Outpatient in a bed. Huron Consulting.

Zelem, J. (2018). Making Sense of it All: The Varying Terms and Definitions Case Managers Face Every Day RACMonitor. https://racmonitor.com/making-sense-of-it-all-the-varying-terms-and-definitions-case-managers-face-every-day/#:%20%20%20~:text=Observation%20Services%2C%20restated%20in%20Transmittal,or%20ways%20to%20classify%20patients

Resources

Medicare Policy Manual https://www.cms.gov/Regulations-and-Guidance/Guidance/Manuals/Internet-Only-Manuals-IOMs-Items/CMS012673

Varying Terms and Definitions Article https://racmonitor.com/making-sense-of-it-all-the-varying-terms-and-definitions-case-managers-face-every-day/#:%20%20%20~:text=Observation%20Services%2C%20restated%20in%20Transmittal,or%20ways%20to%20classify%20patients

LENGTH OF STAY MANAGEMENT

Hospitals face tremendous challenges to stay viable and continue to serve the patients in their communities. It is imperative that hospitals operate as efficiently as possible include because there are many external sources of pressure that threaten financial viability such as:

- Aging populations living longer with multiple comorbidities
- Federal focus on healthcare, leading to reduction in payments for care rendered
- Increases in uninsured populations due to economic downturns
- Increasing prices from suppliers
- Complex and costly healthcare technology advances

Background

Inpatient length of stay (LOS) is one of the biggest issues facing hospitals today. The longer a patient stays in the hospital, there is a greater risk that they will develop a healthcare-acquired infection (HAI).

New research demonstrates that one in five patients who stay a week in hospital will acquire an infection during their stay. The study titled *How dangerous is a day in hospital?* found that a one-night hospital stay carried a 3.4% risk of experiencing an adverse drug reaction, an 11.1% risk of acquiring an infection, and a 0.4% chance of an getting a pressure injury (Agency for Healthcare Research and Quality (AHRQ), 2016).

For a five-night stay, this risk increased to a 5.5% chance of a drug reaction, a 17.6% chance of a hospital-acquired infection, and a 3.1% chance of a pressure injury. A seven-night stay carried a 6.1% chance of an adverse reaction to a drug because of an error or unknown allergy and a 2.5% chance of a pressure ulcer from not being moved enough (AHRQ, 2016).

On average, every additional day in hospital increased the probability of suffering an adverse drug event by about 0.5%, infection by 1.6%, and pressure injury by 0.5%. Reducing hospital LOS is a primary indicator of a hospital's success in achieving patient care quality and safety goals because it avoids unnecessary hospital-acquired conditions (HACs) (AHRQ, 2016).

Hospitals also benefit from a shorter LOS, in that, the facility does not have to cover the expense of treating a HAI and there is a demonstrated decrease in the risk of complications. Additionally, more effective patient LOS management improves patient throughput, enabling the hospital to serve more patients and maximizes reimbursement.

The average length of stay (ALOS) in a hospital is used to gauge the efficiency of a healthcare facility. The most recent figures reported demonstrate the national average for a hospital stay is 4.5

days with the average cost of $10,400 per day (AHRQ, 2019). U.S. hospital stays cost the health system at least $377.5 billion per year. In today's value-based care environment, hospitals are under increasing pressure to avoid patient harm and maintain quality while also lowering costs.

History

Years ago, when you stayed in the hospital, the hospital would send a bill to Medicare or your insurance company that included charges for every band-aid, x-ray, alcohol swab, bedpan, and aspirin, as well as a room charge for each day you were in the hospital. This billing model encouraged hospitals to keep you hospitalized for as long as possible and to provide as many services and products as possible while you were in the hospital. After all, the longer you were in the hospital, the more money the hospital made on room and other charges. The more procedures you had done while hospitalized, the more supplies used. However, as healthcare costs went up, the government sought a way to control costs while encouraging hospitals to provide care more efficiently.

How We Get Paid

Hospitals get paid by Medicare, Medicaid, and third-party payers (insurance companies) based on a formula that includes several elements. The formula is specific to categories of diagnoses referred to as Diagnosis Related Groups (DRGs).

The payment for the DRGs are predetermined. The amount doesn't change regardless of the cost of care. The only way for hospitals to stay in business is to provide care for the patient in a manner that is medically appropriate to efficiently move the patient safely out of the hospital, while keeping the cost below the amount of the DRG payment. If the cost to provide care for the patient exceeds the reimbursement payment, then the hospital will lose money on that case.

Costs come in many forms. Every test, treatment, meal, and room cleaning service costs money. Most hospitals can estimate a cost of $500-$2,000 for an average day in the hospital. Alone that cost may be tolerable. However, this can lead to a large amount accumulating over the course of a year. This is why there is such a focus on keeping LOS to a minimum.

Starting in the 1980s, DRGs changed how Medicare pays hospitals. Instead of paying for each day in the hospital and every individual supply used for care, Medicare pays a single amount for the hospitalization based on the DRG. The DRG is determined by the patient's diagnosis (including secondary diagnosis, if applicable), any surgical procedures performed, and age, and gender. Each DRG encompasses patients who have clinically similar diagnoses, and whose care requires a similar amount of resources to treat. The DRG system is intended to essentially equalize hospital profit margins, regardless of where a hospital is or what type of patients it treats.

Inpatient LOS & DRG Impact

To know how we are doing, we need a standard for comparison. Medicare generally tracks and reports LOS as a "Geometric Mean Length of Stay" or GMLOS. Almost all healthcare entities from hospitals to insurance companies use the Medicare data as their standard for comparison.

GMLOS is calculated by multiplying all of the lengths of stay and then taking the 'nth' root of that number. So why does Medicare use the GMLOS? The advantage of the GMLOS is that it will minimize the impact of outliers. If the number of patients used to calculate the average LOS (ALOS) is relatively low, one patient with an uncharacteristically long or short LOS will significantly increase or decrease the ALOS respectively, but the effect on the GMLOS will be less dramatic. Medicare determines the appropriate LOS based on a large amount of data that includes outliers on both extremes. The goal is to get to a number that can be utilized in the DRG payment formula. In my opinion, GMLOS at this time, is the best method for that purpose.

Using the GMLOS as the goal LOS, the professional case manager communicates and works proactively with all healthcare team members to provide quality care in a more efficient timeline.

Let's take an example of a patient admitted for chronic obstructive pulmonary disease (COPD) without complication or comorbidity (CC) or major complication or comorbidity (MCC). The average cost of actual care for a three-day admission (all cost inclusive) is approximately $28,000 at a local facility.

The total reimbursement based on the Medicare DRG for COPD is $4,807.62. This is not the amount of reimbursement per day, but rather for the entire episode reimbursement. This would include room and board, nursing care, medications, treatments, therapies, and more. The reimbursement is inclusive of all services the patient received while in the hospital.

- Managing LOS yields the following results:
    - 3-day LOS is $1,602.54 per day
    - 7-day LOS is $686.80 per day
    - 10-day LOS is $480.76 per day

Medicaid payment (Illinois in this case) is substantially lower at $2,594.85 total reimbursement for COPD under DRG 192. The amount paid per day is the total reimbursement amount divided by the actual LOS to determine the reimbursement per day. Managing the Medicaid LOS becomes more critical as the "pot of money" can be substantially lower. For example, a diganosis of COPD without CC or MCC, a 3 day LOS calculates to $864.95/day; 7 day LOS yields $370.69/day and 10 day LOS, $259.48 in reimbursement per day.

Medicaid payment is set by the individual state, as Medicaid is a state administered health plan. To illustrate the differences, let's look at the same diagnosis (COPD without CC/MCC, DRG 192) in California.

The same DRG COPD (192) under Medi-Cal (California Medicaid) pays $3,990.00. Similar to the Illinois example, the simple math of reimbursement divided by length of stay notes how the one-time payment can be significantly decreased as the length of stay increases versus actual cost of care. A 3-day LOS divides out to $1,330.00 per day; a 7-day LOS, $570.00 per day and a 10-day LOS yields $399.00 per day. Just as in Illinois, this information is readily accessible through the California Department of Health Care Services website (CA.gov, 2020). *See Example 2.1 on page 40.*

The opportunity to reduce the risk of harm to patients from extended LOS while significantly reduce costs is demonstrated by an example given by Kaufman, Hall and Associates (2019). In this example, the "excess day opportunity" is defined as the difference between the GMLOS and the actual LOS. It is calculated by subtracting the population or overall GMLOS from the actual population or overall LOS for the same time period. The resulting number is the "excess days opportunity." This information can be used to identify areas of opportunity for improvement and can be sorted or broken down by practitioner, service line or department.

Focus Area	Low	Medium	High
Percent Improvement	25%	40%	55%
Excess Day Opportunity	11,500	18,400	25,300
Potential additional bed capacity per day	32	50	69
Cost of additional day ($500 cost reduction per day excess day opportunity)	$5,750,000	$9,200,000	$12,650,000

Table 2.1 Length of stay opportunity
Adapted from Kaufman, Hall and Associates (2019). Table layout by author.

Example 2.1

A simplified version goes like this: Mr. Koff and Mr. Flemm were both admitted to the same hospital for treatment of COPD.

- Mr. Koff was treated and released in two days.
- Mr. Flemm's hospitalization lasted 10 days.

Since Mr. Koff and Mr. Flemm have the same diagnosis, they have the same DRG.

- Based on that DRG, Medicare pays the hospital the same amount for Mr. Koff as it does for Mr. Flemm, even though the hospital spent more money providing 10 days of care to Mr. Flemm than providing two days of care to Mr. Koff.

With a DRG, Medicare pays for a hospitalization based on the diagnosis the patient was hospitalized to treat, NOT based on

- how much the hospital did to treat the patient
- how long the patient was hospitalized
- how much the hospital spent caring for the patient.

In the case of Mr. Koff, the hospital may have made a small profit. The DRG-based payment was probably a little bit larger than the actual cost of Mr. Koff's two-day stay.

In the case of Mr. Flemm, the hospital probably lost money. It surely cost the hospital more to care for Mr. Flemm for 10 days than the DRG-based payment it received.

https://www.verywellhealth.com/drg-101

Best Practices

Daily Multidisciplinary Rounds (MDR)

The care team meets to discuss every patient, every day. This approach promotes interdisciplinary collaboration. As described by Karen Zander (2010), the conversation is very structured and addresses the following information.

I. Plan for the Way
- Physician's plan of care

II.　Plan for the Day
- Interdisciplinary team plan of care for the patient on a given day

III.　Plan for the Stay
- The professional case manager provides an overview of the stay and what is happening today to achieve discharge as close as possible to GMLOS

IV.　Plan for the Pay
- The case manager gives an update on the plan to assure the hospital received payment for services AND the patient can access funding for post discharge plans

---

In a nutshell, the MDR should address and answer these four questions:

- Why is the patient here?
- What are we doing about why the patient is here?
- How will we know when this patient is ready for discharge?
- Are there any barriers to discharge and what are we doing to address them?

Weekly: Extended LOS Review

The case management team convenes a weekly review to discuss cases with "extended lengths of stay." These could be current, in-house patients and/or discharged patients being reviewed retrospectively. The extended day threshold is set by the team and can be lowered as process improvements decrease the average length of stay. The goal is, through discussion of the individual cases, to identify barriers, track avoidable days, and look for trends to create solutions and bring awareness of issues.

An example would be in the discussion of a patient with a 6-day length of stay, identifying the admitting complaint was "chest pain" and the patient had been awaiting cardiology testing (stress test, echocardiogram and potential cardiac catheterization) over a holiday weekend, resulting in a minimum delay of three (3) days due to lack of diagnostic testing over the holiday weekend.

Focus on Flow/Throughput Management

Throughput is the key in a healthcare facility. Moving patients efficiently and effectively along the internal care continuum is a vital part of the professional case manager's role and contributes to decreasing the LOS. Careful mapping of how patients flow through the hospital and into other outside systems, plus a clear understanding of the operational processes behind the flow are two successful approaches to reducing LOS. Success is the result of multiple complementary changes, including both the design of how patients flow through the system and the development of efficient new care delivery models.

Conclusion

Get the basics right from the start. Build a base of success from the time the patient enters your care. These basics include:

- Discharge planning assessment started at the time of admission
- Actively identifying potentially complex discharges
- Setting patient and caregiver expectations by clearly communicating a predicted date of discharge based on GMLOS data
- Creating standardized pathways for common patient types that are based on evidence and clinical consensus
- Proactive end-of-life planning discussions
- Ensuring good communication for smooth handovers and transitions

Bundle approaches together. No single approach will achieve sustained reductions in LOS. Approaches should include a focus on the internal and external care continuums, including internal hospital flow and alternative out-of-hospital provision with the main goal of increasing patient safety and outcomes. Case managers should look for efficiencies such as:

- Non-life-threatening issues that can be addressed as an outpatient status or followed up at the physician's office following discharge
- Reducing routine screening tests that are not related to the reason for admission (mammogram, routine colonoscopy)
- Ensure active support for discharge seven days a week. Several factors contributing to unnecessarily prolonged LOS are more pronounced at weekends, such as variable staffing and service levels in hospitals and variable access to community services

A collaborative approach and use of best practice management processes ensure that every patient receives the right care, in the right setting, at the right time—every time. Managing inpatient LOS is a means of enhancing patient throughput, improving patient safety and experience, decreasing HAI risks, and augmenting the financial picture for the facility to ensure the facility is there to serve the next patient.

References

6 ways hospitals can reduce length of stays. (2013). FierceHealthcare.

AHRQ (2016). Length of stay reduction and management.

AHRQ (2019). Length of stay reduction and management update.

Bethea, D., Holland Jr., C., Reddick, B. (2014). Storming the gates of interprofessional collaboration. *Nursing Management, 45*(9).

CA.gov (2020). Department of Health Care Services. DRG Pricing Resources for SFY 2020/21.

Case Management Society of America. (2016). Case Management Standards of Practice.

Centers for Medicare and Medicaid. (2017). DRG Calculator.

Communicating for success (2018). CCMC IssueBrief, April 2018.

Davis, E. (2020). Diagnostic related grouping and how it works.

Lamb, G., (2015). Overview and Summary: Care Coordination: Benefits of Interprofessional Collaboration. *The Online Journal of Issues in Nursing, 20*(3).

Lewis, R & Edwards, N (2015). *Improving length of stay: What can hospitals do?* Nuffield Trust, September 2015.

Pisarsky, B. & Pike, T. (2019). *A new look at length of stay.* Kaufman, Hall & Associates

Reducing length of stay improves outcomes. (2018). Health Catalyst.

Stark, J., (2010). Top 10 hospital case manager best practices. *Case Management Monthly*, November 2010.

State of Illinois. (2020). Illinois Medicaid EAPG Pricing Calculator. Accessed July 13, 2021.

Zander, K., (2010). Case Management accountability for safe, smooth and sustained transitions. *Professional Case Management, 15*(4).

Resources

Illinois Medicaid Reimbursement Calculator https://www.illinois.gov/hfs/SiteCollectionDocuments/ILEAPGCalculatorEff20200701EXTERNALBild20200827.xlsx

California Medicaid Reimbursement Calculator California Department of Health Care Services website at https://www.dhcs.ca.gov/provgovpart/Pages/DRG-Pricing-Resources-for-SFY-202021.aspx

OBSERVATION VERSUS INPATIENT COMPARISON

Anna Rheka Winkowski MSN RN CCM ACM-RN

It is not uncommon for patients to assume that they are admitted as an inpatient when they spend a night or two in the hospital. Why? Because they get assigned a hospital bed, they are receiving care like everyone else, and they get served hospital food. When the case manager shows up with the Medicare Outpatient Observation Notification letter (also known as a MOON letter), patients get a little perturbed, especially when they read the part about being responsible for the co-pays.

Observation Status Defined

What exactly is an observation status and how is it any different from an inpatient status? CMS defines observation status as "a status commonly assigned to patients who present to the emergency department and who then require a significant period of treatment or monitoring before a decision is made concerning their admission or discharge" (Medicare Benefit Policy, 2005). The purpose of placing a patient in an observation status is to monitor whether there is an improvement in the patient's condition within 24-48 hours or whether further tests or treatment are needed, thereby requiring an inpatient admission (Medicare Benefit Policy, 2005).

Medicare Part B is responsible for paying most of the physician charges when the patient is in an observation status. The patient is responsible for 20% of the Medicare-approved charges after paying their Part B deductible, as well as the copayment for each of the outpatient services they receive while hospitalized (Are you Hospital Inpatient or Outpatient?, 2018). As a case manager, your role is to be able to articulate to the patient and their caregiver what it means to be assigned an observation status because the minute your patient hears about their financial responsibility, they can either ask to be discharged or they will ask their physician to change their status to inpatient, even if it may not be appropriate.

Inpatient Status

A patient is in an inpatient status when the physician determines the patient will require two or more nights of medically necessary hospital stay, and a formal order for an inpatient stay is entered in the patient's medical record. Medicare Part A generally pays for the hospitalization. This explains why some patients would ask their physician to change their status to inpatient once they find out they are in observation status. Being an inpatient is important because Medicare requires that a patient has qualifying hospital stay to be eligible to go to a skilled nursing facility (SNF). What is considered a "qualifying hospital stay"? A patient must have three consecutive inpatient days, excluding the day of discharge, for Medicare to cover a short-term SNF stay following discharge.

As a case manager, you must be vigilant of physicians who will enter an order for inpatient stay to qualify the patient for a SNF stay. Your Utilization Review Nurse must review the patient's chart using your facility's tool to determine whether an admission is appropriate for inpatient status or not. It is crucial the review is done in a timely manner as an overnight stay while the patient is still in observation status will not count towards the qualifying stay for SNF services. This happens because the inpatient stay only becomes official once the physician enters a formal order for inpatient stay. It's important to have your Physician Advisor and/or Case Management Director involved when you have a physician who constantly tries to admit a patient inappropriately. Their input is essential to avoid any issues which could result in financial penalties or worse, citations down the line.

How do you know when a patient should be observation versus inpatient?

Observation	Inpatient
Usually "symptom-driven" diagnosis or "rule out"	Usually have a defined "disease" diagnosis
Expected to improve within 24 hours	Patient will be unlikely ready for discharge within 24 hours
Diagnostic procedures ordered are usually done as outpatient	Treatment required can only be provided in acute hospital setting
Order should clearly state: "Place in observation status"	Order should clearly state: "Admit as inpatient"

Table 2.2 Observation vs. Inpatient Status
Adapted from Centers for Medicare and Medicaid (n.d.) Table design by author.

Below are examples of patient scenarios from Medicare.gov (Inpatient or Outpatient Hospital Status Affects Your Cost, n.d.), which shows what services are covered by Part A and what services are covered by Part B. Your patient will still be responsible for any deductible, coinsurance, and copayment as outlined by Medicare.

Situation: Patient is in the Emergency Department (ED) (also known as the Emergency Room or "ER") and then formally admitted to the hospital with a doctor's order.

Inpatient vs. Outpatient
Outpatient until patient is formally admitted as an inpatient based on the doctor's order. Inpatient after admission.

Part A Payment
Patient's inpatient hospital stay, and all related outpatient services provided during the 3 days before the admission date.

Part B Payment
Physician services or "pro fees"

Situation: Patient comes to the ED with chest pain, and the hospital keeps him/her for 2 nights. One night is spent in observation and the doctor writes an order for inpatient admission on the second day.

Inpatient vs. Outpatient
Outpatient until formally admitted as an inpatient based on the doctor's order. Inpatient after admission.

Part A Payment
Patient's inpatient hospital stay, and all related outpatient services provided during the 3 days before the admission date.

Part B Payment
Physician services or "pro fees"

Situation: Patient presents to a hospital for outpatient surgery, but was kept overnight due to elevated blood pressure. The doctor doesn't write an order to admit as an inpatient. Patient returns home the next day.

Inpatient vs. Outpatient
Outpatient

Part A Payment
Nothing

Part B Payment
Physician services and hospital outpatient services (for example, surgery, lab tests, or intravenous medicines)

Situation: The physician writes an order for the patient to be admitted as an inpatient. However, after chart review by the UR RN, it was determined the patient's hospital status is appropriate for observation. The physician must agree, and the patient must be told in writing before discharge that their hospital status was changed from inpatient to outpatient.

Inpatient vs. Outpatient
Outpatient

Part A Payment
Nothing

Part B Payment
Physician services and hospital outpatient services

References

Centers for Medicare and Medicaid. (2005). Pub 100-02 Medicare benefit policy.

Centers for Medicare and Medicaid. (n.d.). Are you a hospital inpatient or outpatient?

Centers for Medicare and Medicaid. (n.d.). Inpatient or outpatient hospital status affects your costs.

Resources

Are you a hospital inpatient or outpatient? https://www.medicare.gov/sites/default/files/2018-09/11435-Are-You-an-Inpatient-or-Outpatient.pdf

Inpatient or outpatient hospital status affects your costs. https://www.medicare.gov/what-medicare-covers/what-part-a-covers/inpatient-or-outpatient-hospital-status

Medicare benefit policy. https://www.cms.gov/Regulations-and-Guidance/Guidance/Manuals/Internet-Only-Manuals-IOMs-Items/CMS012673

CMS INPATIENT ONLY LIST (IPO)

Anna Rheka Winkowski MSN RN CCM ACM-RN

In 2001, CMS created the Hospital Outpatient Prospective Payment System (OPPS), which established services that could be provided safely to Medicare patients in an outpatient setting. CMS also created an Inpatient Only List (IPO), which is published every year on November 1st and is updated annually in the OPPS Final Rule. The Medicare IPO identifies services and procedures (about 1,700 procedures) that are typically provided in an inpatient setting and are not paid in OPPS. Most of the services on the list are surgical procedures considered complicated and would require post-recovery care for at least 24 hours in an inpatient setting.

Sounds easy, right? If you are a novice case manager, you are probably thinking just give me the list and I will make sure if the procedure is on the IPO, we will have the physician enter an inpatient order, use the justification the procedure is in the IPO and we are good to go! Not so fast. If you are a seasoned case manager reading this, you are probably thinking it is not as black and white as they make it sound and you are correct!

The Reality

Too often, you have a patient coming in for a knee replacement (CPT 27447), which is not on the IPO, but your physician indicates the patient will need an inpatient stay. As a case manager, do you insist the physician keeps the patient as an outpatient because the procedure is not on the IPO? No. As a case manager, your role first and foremost, is to be an advocate for the patient. When you get in situations like this, you review the History and Physical and speak to the physician. The patient could have an underlying condition that would require close monitoring post-operatively. Perhaps the patient has pain issues. Documentation is key to support the patient's admission status and developing a relationship with your outpatient (OP) surgery team is important. Why? If the physician does not want to speak to you, the OP surgery team can help you get the information you need or convey necessary information to the physician.

On the other hand, you could have a patient whose procedure is listed on the IPO, but the physician indicates the patient is being discharged later that day. You must make sure the procedure is in fact on the IPO and an inpatient order is entered even if the patient is getting discharged that same day. Why is that? Without an order for the inpatient stay, the hospital will not be able to bill for their service. The hospital will not be able to bill for an outpatient stay either because the procedure is listed in the IPO. I know it can be confusing! While you are responsible for advocating for your patients, you also must be a good steward for your facility's resources. Someone has to pay the bills, right?

Addendum E

Table 2.3 Inpatient Only Procedures provides an example of a list of inpatient only procedures for 2021, which means that anytime a patient has one of the procedures performed from the list, it meets the criteria for an inpatient admission (CMS Inpatient Only List, 2021). Addendum E is an excel file that lists Healthcare Common Procedure Coding System or HCPCS codes only payable as inpatient procedures (CMS1204971, 2021).

HCPCS Code	Procedure	HCPCS Code	Procedure
31760	Repair of windpipe	33425	Repair of mitral valve
38102	Removal of spleen total	33535	CABG Artery x 3
43360	Gastrointestinal repair	43846	Gastric bypass for obesity
50075	Removal of kidney stone	58150	Total hysterectomy
55821	Removal of prostate	47610	Removal of gallbladder

Table 2.3 Inpatient Only Procedures
Adapted from Centers for Medicare and Medicaid (2021). Table design by author.

As a CM, you are not expected to remember all of the HCPCS or Current Procedural Terminology or CPT codes. However, some of will become familiar over time because they are done frequently. There cannot be enough emphasis placed on the importance of having a relationship with the OP surgery team.

Best practices include:

- Have the OP surgery team fax the weekly surgical schedule for the CM team to review and flag CPT codes that are on the IPO

- Have the daily surgical schedule faxed twice: first thing in the morning and in the afternoon for the next day's schedule, to ensure that CM has reviewed the CPT codes for the add-on surgeries.

- Have someone from the CM team reviewing this list and immediately reaching out to the OP surgery team if there is a CPT code that is on the IPO with the admission status entered as outpatient.
  - They HAVE to match, or your facility will not be able to bill for that service. The physicians will get paid under Medicare Part B, but the facility will not be able to get paid under Medicare Part A if there is not an order for an inpatient stay.
    › Note that "removal of gallbladder" is currently on the IPO list but if the IPO HCPCS code is not the correct classification for the surgery performed, the case will not be coded or paid as IPO. A majority of gallbladder removals are done as outpatient, laparoscopic procedures. Validating the post-procedure codes is a must.

The Latest

In August 2020, CMS proposed policies aimed at increasing choice, lowering patient's out-of-pocket costs, empowering patients, and protecting taxpayer dollars (Newsroom Fact Sheet, 2020). One of those policies is phasing out the IPO over three years starting in calendar year (CY) 2021 with the list completely phased out by CY 2024. CMS proposed the removal of over 300 musculoskeletal-related procedures from the IPO, making them eligible for Medicare to pay in the hospital outpatient setting (Newsroom Fact Sheet, 2020). Once removed from the IPO, procedures will be subject to the two-midnight rule after the two-year exemption expires. During the two-year period, Beneficiary Family Centered Care-Quality Improvement Organization (BFCC-QIO) will review the short-stay inpatient claims of those procedures recently removed from the IPO, for medical necessity and educate providers on the two-midnight rule.

So, why go on and on about IPO if it is going to be phased out anyway? Because until it is totally phased out, CM is still responsible for ensuring the IPO is being followed.

Most of what is in the IPO list are complex surgical procedures that require patients to stay in the hospital as an inpatient, for at least 24 hours or more, for post-operative recovery. In December 2020, CMS released the final OPPS rule which would phase out the IPO list over a period of three years beginning in January 2021 and ending in December 2024. While 300 musculoskeletal-related procedures are removed from the list, acute facilities are still responsible for making sure the remaining procedures in the IPO list are being assigned the correct admission status of inpatient.

Update as of July 2021:

In an unprecedented move, the Centers for Medicare & Medicaid Services (CMS) has proposed in the 2022 Outpatient Prospective Payment System (OPPS) Rule to put back on the inpatient only list all the procedures that they removed from the inpatient only list starting this calendar year (Buck, 2021).

CMS has also put the brakes on its plan to completely eliminate the inpatient only list. As we know, change is ever present in the healthcare world. This particular topic illustrates this point very clearly and the importance of the professional case manager staying current on issues that impact our practice.

References

Buck, C. (2021). Breaking news: CMS to reinstate Inpatient Only List. www.icd10monitor.com

Centers for Medicare and Medicaid Services. (2021). Hospital Inpatient PPS.

Centers for Medicare and Medicaid Services. (2020). Newsroom Fact Sheet.

Resources

Hospital Inpatient PPS. https://www.cms.gov/Medicare/Medicare-Fee-for-Service-Payment/AcuteInpatientPPS#:~:text=This%20payment%20system%20is%20referred,Medicare%20patients%20in%20that%20DRG

CONDITION CODE 44

Definition

Changing the status of Medicare patients per guidelines described in Condition 44, Transmittal 299 of the Medicare Manual. Transmittal 299 summarizes the requirements that this change in patient status will require use of Condition Code 44, which is described as "inpatient admission changed to observation." In some instances, a physician may order inpatient services, but upon internal utilization review and before claim submission, the facility may determine the services do not meet inpatient criteria.

Background

CMS created Condition Code 44 to address occasions where an admission occurs when there is not a case manager on duty to offer guidance, when internal review determines that an inpatient admission does not meet hospital criteria, or when a patient would have usually been registered as an outpatient. Prior to implementation of Condition Code 44, a hospital could only bill or receive payment for certain services under Medicare Part B if the retrospective review failed for payment as inpatient status under Medicare Part A payment (self-deny the bill or claim). Condition Code 44 allows hospitals to retroactively correct the status prior to discharge and treat the entire episode of care as an outpatient encounter, enabling payment for services from the date of admission rather than date of status order change.

The following methodology outlines the framework to determine the change in patient admission status from inpatient to observation for Medicare patients and the procedure for billing and applying the Condition Code 44 process. Under the Utilization Management Conditions of Participation, using Condition Code 44, the Utilization Review Committee (URC) may change the patient status to outpatient provided the following conditions are met:

- The hospital has not submitted a claim to Medicare for the inpatient admission
- The Attending Physician agrees with the Utilization Review Physician Advisor's (URPA) decision or two physician members of the URC overrule the attending physician's disagreement
- The attending physician's agreement with the utilization review URPA's decision or the determination of the URC physician members and is documented in the patient's medical record
- The change in patient status from inpatient to outpatient is made prior to discharge or release, while the patient is still the hospital, prior to a discharge order being written

Case Manager's Role

A professional case manager, who is a non-physician member of the URC, reviews Medicare inpatients utilizing the facility's contracted and preferred medical decision-making criteria for medical necessity of the admission to an Inpatient status.

If, after reviewing a Medicare inpatient record, the case manager (CM) determines the clinical documentation does not meet InterQual criteria for inpatient level of care, the CM will contact the URPA with their findings. The case manager requests the physician advisor to review the case and issue a recommendation to determine the appropriate status.

If the medical facts and documentation are in concurrence (agreement) with URPA the patient does not meet criteria for inpatient status, the CM will notify the attending physician. The attending physician will review the findings and recommendation from the URPA, potentially securing concurrence with the findings.

If the attending physician concurs with the non-inpatient status, the CM documents this conversation per facility protocols noting the attending physician concurs with the URPA the "patient does not meet criteria for inpatient status and the patient status is changed from inpatient to observation." This must be written prior to the patient's discharge.

If the attending physician disagrees, the case will be referred to at least two additional physicians who include either a physician member of the URC, or the department chair. If two of these physicians agree with the CM and URPA's findings, the agreement is documented, and the patient's status is changed from inpatient to observation. If the attending physician refuses to write the status change order, the order will be written by one of the two physicians involved in the decision changing the patient's status.

Case management will document the corresponding Code 44 condition code along with the date and time of the change. The change must be fully documented in the medical record to include:

- Orders (updated, signed, and dated by the physician).
- Notes that indicate why the change was made.
- Care that was furnished to the beneficiary.
- Participants in making decision to change the patient's status.

Patient Impact

The patient must be notified in writing of the change and any impact on his/her financial liability. CMS states that "Medicare beneficiaries have the right to participate in treatment decisions and to know their treatment choices. They are also entitled to receive information about co-insurance and deductibles" (MLN Matters, SE0622, 2004). Requiring that a change in patient status be made before the patient is discharged ensures the patient is fully informed about the status change and its impact on the co-insurance and deductible for which the beneficiary would be responsible. This aligns closely with the CM's advocate role for the patient and the "right care, right setting, right time" mantra of case management.

References

Centers for Medicare and Medicaid. (2004). Medicare Claims Processing Manual, Condition Code 44.

Centers for Medicare and Medicaid. (2004). MLN Matters SE0622, Clarification of Medicare Payment Policy When Inpatient Admission Is Determined Not To Be Medically Necessary, Including the Use of Condition Code 44: "Inpatient Admission Changed to Outpatient". September 2004.

Hirsch, R. (2015). 11 things to know about Condition Code 44. Becker's Hospital Review, September 2015

Resource

Condition Code 44 Guidance https://www.cms.gov/regulations-and-guidance/guidance/transmittals/downloads/r299cp.pdf

DISCHARGE DISPOSITION

A patient discharge status code is a two-digit code that identifies where the patient is at the conclusion of a healthcare facility encounter or at the end of a billing cycle. The discharge status code identifies where the patient is being discharged to at the end of their facility stay or transferred to such as an acute/post-acute facility (Center for Medicare and Medicaid, 2019). Table 2.4 provides a selection of commonly used discharge disposition codes.

The discharging facility should ensure the discharge code used is correct and the patient's medical record supports the discharge status code used. Use of an incorrect code may affect the facility's payment, but will impact any other service receiving the patient, often preventing them from successfully submitting their claim (Besler, 2020).

01	Discharge to Home
02	Discharged/Transferred to Short Term General Hospital
03	Discharged/Transferred to Skilled Nursing Facility (SNF)
04	Discharged/Transferred to Intermediate Care Facility (ICF)
06	Discharged/Transferred to Home Health Care Services (HHC)
07	Left Against Medical Advice (AMA)
20	Expired
21	Discharged/Transferred to Court/Law Enforcement
43	Discharged/Transferred to Federal Hospital, VA Hospital
50	Discharged/Transferred to Hospice/ Home
51	Discharged/Transferred to Hospice, Inpatient
62	Discharged/Transferred to Inpatient Rehabilitation Facility (IRF)
63	Discharged/Transferred to Long Term Acute Care Hospital (LTACH)
65	Discharged/Transferred to Psychiatric Facility

Table 2.4 Commonly used discharge disposition codes
Adapted from Center for Medicare and Medicaid (2019). Table design by author.

Example 2.2

Mr. Smith is discharged to home with home health services. The CM incorrectly selects Discharge Disposition 01 (discharge to a home/self-care) instead of the correct Discharge Disposition 06 (home with home health services).

Implications

Selecting an incorrect discharge disposition or not reconciling the discharge disposition post-discharge could impact the ability for the hospital and any post-acute provider to receive the appropriate payment for services rendered. In this example, the home health care agency's claim would be rejected.

Incorrect discharge dispositions can lead to underpayments, overpayments subject to recovery, or the post-acute provider having claims rejected if the discharge disposition does not indicate transition to post-acute services.

Best Practices

The professional CM should ensure the correct discharge disposition code is assigned at the time of discharge. Clearly documenting the final discharge disposition in the case management notes and providing education to those team members that may be entering discharge disposition codes into the medical record system on where to find this information for their reference is vital. Processes to validate the discharge disposition post-discharge should also be in place for billing reconciliation purposes.

References

Center for Medicare and Medicaid. (2019). Patient discharge codes matter.

HCPro. (2010). Don't let improper discharge disposition codes fly under the radar at your facility.

Resources

Patient discharge codes. https://www.cms.gov/Outreach-and-Education/Medicare-Learning-Network-MLN/MLNMattersArticles/downloads/SE1411.pdf

UTILIZATION MANAGEMENT TOOLS

"You're only as good as the tools you use." This saying has been around for many years and highlights the importance of using the correct tool for the job. Tools in case management? While we may not use a hammer, saw or screwdrivers, we do use a variety of tools to get the job done. Devices, equipment, software, resources, applications, workflows—tools can be anything that is utilized during the job to assist you in completing the elements of your work. Some of the tools used in the Utilization Management side of case management include: CMS's UR CoP resources (See Chapter 1), medical necessity criteria, review templates, and other "cheat sheets" that can be used to educate or reference for streamlining the work process.

Medical Necessity

Medical necessity is the cornerstone of Utilization Management (UM), which is defined as "healthcare services or supplies that are needed to diagnose or treat an illness, injury, condition, disease, or its symptoms – and that meet accepted standards of medicine" (CMS, 2018). The process of validating medical necessity for Inpatient level of care include consideration of the following criteria:

- The severity of the patient's presenting symptoms or illness
- The intensity of the interventions given to the patient in response to the patient's presentation and the level of care needed to administer the interventions safely across the progression of care
  - Interventions that are related to and needed for the diagnosis, care, or treatment of the patient's medical condition.
  - Interventions that meet the standards of good medical practice in the local area and are not for the convenience of the patient or their provider.

As defined by CMS, documentation to support medical necessity should support the medical need for the services rendered. The documentation may include evaluations or records from physicians, consultations, progress notes, physician's office, hospital, nursing home, home health agency, other healthcare professionals, and test reports.

Criteria Sets

While medical decision-making is documented in the medical record, healthcare facilities may use a published criteria set to validate medical necessity and provide guidelines for admission, discharge, and movement along the care continuum. "Prior to the general use of consistent and rigorous utilization management, widespread care variations, excessive healthcare costs, and less-than-optimal care were the rule rather than the exception" (Mitus, 2008).

Additionally, most payers apply clinical review information received to a criteria set as a tool to determine medical necessity, authorization or denial of the admission, continued stay, service, or post-acute transitions.

There are several criteria sets that are available commercially, including the two most commonly utilized: InterQual by Change Healthcare and MCG (formerly Milliman Care Guidelines). Healthcare facilities and payers may use a published criteria set, screening guideline, or may develop their own. The CMS Conditions of Participation (CoP) for Utilization Review (482.30(f)) note that "the Utilization Review Committee must review professional services provided, to determine medical necessity and to promote the most efficient use of available health facilities and services" (Centers for Medicare and Medicaid, 2018). The CoP does not state how the utilization review must be carried out nor does it recommend a process or procedure. This is determined by each facility in their Utilization Management Plan. Please note that CMS does not endorse the use of any particular brand of criteria set or screening guidelines. CMS refers back to the Federal Rule that physician decision-making determines whether a patient requires hospital admission what level of care is medically appropriate.

References

Centers for Medicare and Medicaid. (2018). Conditions of Participation for Utilization Management, section 482.30.

Mitus, A. J. (2008). The birth of InterQual. *Professional Case Management, 13*(4), pp. 228-233.

Resources

InterQual by Change Healthcare https://www.changehealthcare.com

MCG (formerly Milliman Care Guidelines) at www.mcg.com

REVIEW TEMPLATES

Templates, like checklists, are tools to help avoid errors in any process. Templates ensure consistency and completeness by providing a concise, thorough picture of the patient's condition. Sample templates for various levels of UR (admission, continued stay, and discharge) are provided as well as demonstration examples on their use.

These template examples were developed by a group of RNs who specialized in Utilization Management as way to create consistency across the work unit when covering for each other. Many thanks to them for their initiative!

Bold headings denote the data subgroups. Italic entries are the patient level-specific information from the medical record. Note the examples employ a "documentation by exception" strategy for laboratory results, medications pertinent to the ongoing hospital level care, and full vital signs with each submission.

The "blank" template is provided with a sample of what a completed review template looks like for each type (admission, continued stay and discharge).

The goal of the use of templates is to provide a standardized framework for reviews. This creates the consistency across covering as mentioned above but also a great opportunity to ensure nothing is missed when creating the review for submission. Use of templates can decrease denials as the case manager gives a full, complete and concise picture of the patient's current status at the time of review submission.

Admission Review Template

Working DX:
Admission Summary:
PMH
VS:
Labs:
Radiology:
Procedures:
Consults: (pending/complete)
Medications:
Diet:
Activity:
PT/OT/ST:
PLOF/Services Received:
Issues impacting transition:
Working DC Plan:

Sample Completed Admission Review Template

Working DX: Pancreatitis

Admission Summary: 52 y/o male recently treated for acute pancreatitis (admitted and discharged 3/20/15), who presents with 8 hours of intermittent abdominal pain. Patient describes the pain as pressure-like and diffuse without radiation. States nothing makes it better or worse. Denies any associated symptoms such as fever, chills, loss of appetite, N/V/D, or changes in his bowel habits. Patient further denies history of gallstones or heavy alcohol consumption, but he does admit to smoking approx. 1/2 PPD.

PMH: pancreatitis

VS: 97.9 63 18 123/78 97%@RA

Labs: RDW 14.7 Lymph% 18.3 Lymph# 1.0 Cl108 CO220 AG 18.3 BUN 8.4 Lipase731 ETOH 15

Radiology: U/S--No Gallstones

Procedures: none planned

Consults: (pending/complete) GI consult pending.

Medications: 0.9 NaCl IVF 1000ml/hr IV q8H Morphine Sulfate 4mg IV once, Zofran 4mg IV once

Diet: NPO

Activity: ad lib

PT/OT/ST: no referral at this time

PLOF/Services Received: from home with family, Independent.

Issues impacting transition: none identified

Working DC Plan: home with family, OP follow up

Continued Stay Review Template

Working DX:
IMPRESSION
SUBJECTIVE:
OBJECTIVE:
VS:
Labs
Imaging:
Procedures:
Consults: (pending/complete)

Medications:
Activity:
PT/OT/ST:
Issues impacting transition:
Working DC Plan:

Sample Completed Continued Stay Template

Working DX: Pneumonia

IMPRESSION

SUBJECTIVE: Patient conscious, alert, responsive, not in pain or distress, afebrile. The patient has been evaluated by Dr. Jones, he is scheduled for chest tube insertion today under fluoroscopy in the operating room. The patient has history of cough productive of clear sputum but no hemoptysis.

OBJECTIVE: On examination, patient is conscious, alert, responsive, not in pain or distress, afebrile. The patient is on two liters of oxygen by nasal cannula.

He is status post left thoracentesis on 3/22 which showed complicated parapneumonic pleural effusion, probably early empyema. The fluid was clear yellow but turbid.

VS: 97.0 88 20 133/70 97% on O24LNC (OXYGEN, 4 LITERS BY NASAL CANNULA)

Labs: White cell count 17,100, hemoglobin 8.8, hematocrit 27.4, MCV 100.9, platelet count 417,000, neutrophils 80%, lymphocytes 20%, monocytes 5% and 0.6% eosinophils. Sodium 139, potassium 4.5, chloride 102, bicarbonate 30, BUN 17, creatinine 1.6. GFR 58.2. Glucose 120, Accu-Chek 190. Calcium 7.8, phosphorus 3.9, magnesium 2.0, bilirubin 0.8, direct 0.7. AST 20, ALT 15, alkaline phosphatase 155. CPK less than 20. Total protein 6.1, albumin 2.5, globulin 3.6. PT 13.7, INR 1.09, PTT 47.6.

Imaging: no new imaging studies

Procedures: chest tube placement 3/22

Consults: (pending/complete) SX, for chest tube insertion

Medications: insulin sliding scale, Levothyroxine, Tylenol, Ceftriaxone, Hydralazine, NPH insulin, Pantoprazole for GI prophylaxis.

Activity: bed rest

PT/OT/ST: no referrals made at this time

Issues impacting transition: none identified

Working DC Plan: home with OP follow-up

Discharge Review Template

Working DX:
Labs:
Imaging:
Procedures:
Consults: (pending/complete)
Medications:
Diet:
Activity:
PT/OT/ST:
Issues impacting transition:
FINAL DC Plan:

Sample Completed Discharge Review Template

Working DX: pancreatitis

Labs: labs WNL at discharge

Imaging: no new imaging studies

Procedures: NGT discontinued

Consults: (pending/complete) GI, Dr Smith; complete. Continues plan of care as outlined

Medications: IVF @100/hr discontinued, Protonix converted to PO, MSO4 4 mg IV q 4 hours prn (received 2 doses in last 24 hours) converted to Norco PO PRN

Diet: diet advanced as tolerated, resumed General Diet

Activity: ad lib

PT/OT/ST: no referrals made at this time

Issues impacting transition: ETOH use, family dynamic

FINAL DC Plan: Transition to INP Substance Abuse Program per patient's request

THE COLLABORATIVE TEAM INVOLVING CASE/UTILIZATION MANAGERS AND PHYSICIAN ADVISORS

Juliet B. Ugarte Hopkins MD CHCQM-PHYADV FABQAURP

The hospital role of physician advisor has no distinct birthday, nor celebrated date of materialization. It is generally recognized that sometime in the late 1990s, physicians in a number of hospitals across the country found themselves stealthily and deftly nudged by their superiors into an administrative role without distinct borders. These physicians were commonly well-established, internal medicine specialists who cared for patients in the hospital setting, but other subspecialties were utilized as well.

What they all had in common was an interest in topics few of their colleagues wished to consider. Some had a particular focus on quality of care, leaning into newly devised measures created to standardize, track, and pinpoint successes or opportunities. Others were insistent on cultivating excellent documentation. Still, others found themselves drawn to financial relationships with health insurance plans and the manner in which their health system was reimbursed for the care provided to patients.

Titles initially revolved around this individual serving as a "medical director" for a specific department. Over time, as areas of focus merged and the emphasis shifted to educating medical staff, the term "physician advisor" came into being. While universally accepted, even today there continues to be some level of dissatisfaction with the term. What is the individual advising about? Does "physician" refer to the person themselves? Or, the person is providing advice to physicians? Many health systems have tried to rectify this problem by adding a qualifier to "physician advisor" such as, Physician Advisor for Case Management or Physician Advisor for Clinical Documentation Integrity.

Any preoccupations with the title of the role were quickly squashed in 2009 when the Recovery Audit Contractor (RAC) program started. Created to review Medicare claims, identify billing errors, and return improper payments back to the Medicare Trust Fund, physician advisors' overall willingness to focus on "the business of medicine" was cast in a new light. A few years later on October 1, 2013, when the Medicare Two-Midnight Rule came into being, physician advisors' critical role within hospitals and health systems across the country was solidified. Not only was an overall understanding of patient status, medical necessity, hospital service utilization, and comprehensive clinical documentation needed, but the practicing providers also required education to meet a basic level of comprehension and compliance.

The focus of a physician advisor can be singular or broad reaching. According to the 2019 Physician Advisor Survey published by the American College of Physician Advisors (ACPA) (involving 170 respondents from across the United States), the following areas are commonly addressed:

1. Second-level utilization reviews for patient status
2. Leading/supporting Care Management and/or Utilization Management Departments
3. Performing insurance denial appeals
4. Leading/supporting denials management teams
5. Quality projects such as length of stay, core measures, readmissions, patient safety, etc.
6. Clinical documentation integrity and/or coding departments or teams
7. Leading/participating in multi-disciplinary rounds
8. Revenue cycle activities
9. Health information management and/or information technology activities
10. Quality department activities
11. Payor contracting activities
12. Leading and/or supporting compliance
13. Population health

This comprehensive list is daunting in and of itself, but even more so when taking into account that 30% of health systems in which the respondents work have only a single physician advisor on staff and 50% of all respondents still work clinically part-time (American Academy of Physician Advisors, 2020). These limitations lead many hospitals and health systems to silo their physician advisors into addressing a select few of the categories above due to lack of bandwidth. Chief executive officers and chief medical officers with insight and a keen eye on the future recognize the need for increased resources, evolving their programs to create multiple physician advisor positions covering the wide range of topics in which they can provide support.

Focusing on the role of physician advisors in Case Management and Utilization Management truly brings us to the heart of the position itself. Why? In very few other instances does the physician advisor serve as such a champion, educator, mentor, and even confidant to the other professionals in the department. Basic collaboration between physician advisors and case/utilization managers involves – at minimum – a general sense of trust and collegiality which allows for bi-directional flow of queries, direction, and advice.

If case managers feel some questions or situations are somehow beneath a level of importance or significance to escalate to their physician advisor, opportunities will be missed, and errors will be made. Likewise, the full picture of the issue at hand might be missed if a physician advisor does not appreciate the wisdom associated with the extensive experience case managers have in their interactions with patients, families, and care teams.

Basic Collaboration Between Physician Advisors and Case/Utilization Managers

At baseline, collaboration between physician advisors and their case/utilization management teams involve assessment of patient status including all payors involving any point of time during the hospitalization. If further direction is needed after the chart is reviewed using guidance methods such as MCG or InterQual, a referral is sent to the physician advisor.

Questions requiring assessment by a physician advisor will often vary depending on the patient's payor. As Medicare utilizes the Two-Midnight Rule, guidelines and criteria are less important than the provider's expectation (or not) of the patient requiring at least two midnights of medically necessary care in the hospital. Common referrals for patients covered by fee-for-service Medicare involve whether it's reasonable for a provider to anticipate two midnights or, conversely, for them to place a patient into outpatient status with observation services when they don't anticipate two midnights even if guidelines clearly direct the CM that inpatient status is warranted.

Status assessments for patients covered by Medicare Advantage, managed Medicaid, and commercial plans can frequently confuse and confound due to lack of clear direction about what criteria supports inpatient admission. Without the guidance of the Medicare Two-Midnight Rule, it can be extremely frustrating for CMs to assess a patient in outpatient status receiving observation services who is entering calendar day three or four of hospitalization without meeting MCG, InterQual, or other criteria. In these cases, referral to the physician advisor can lead to identification of issues beyond that of patient status, which brings us to the next aspect of basic collaboration between case managers and physician advisors.

Delays in care and deviation from best practice when it comes to medical management of patients in the hospital setting can be subtle and difficult to identify during documentation review. This is why it's common for such issues to surface following day two of hospitalization when it appears there is little progression with the patient's assessment or plan of care, but inpatient criteria are still not supported based on the patient's condition. In cases like this, referral to the physician advisor can lead not only to direction about status, but also recognition of broader challenges.

Discovering missed opportunities involving diet advancement, pain control, scheduling of advanced imaging studies, and procedures like stress tests, use of oral versus intravenous medications, and timing of consultation by specialists can feel a little like opening up Pandora's box. Continually uncovering, investigating, and breaking down the barriers which lead to these deviations can lead to excellent results.

Once again, if case managers are not comfortable bringing to their physician advisor what may initially feel like a nagging sense that something is not progressing as it should, these opportunities will pass by unaddressed. Intuitive physician advisors will recognize when a delay has occurred without escalation by the case manager and question if the omission was due to reluctance to "question the provider's judgement." If confirmed, this can effectively lead to reassurance for the case manager that such concerns are unwarranted.

Beyond day-to-day patient case assessment and investigation is continual education and reinforcement of compliance concepts associated with the Centers for Medicare and Medicaid Services (CMS) rules and regulations along with contract-specific rules applying to payors contracted with the hospital or health system. As with virtually every other aspect of medicine, the business of healthcare is no different. It's a fool's errand to rely on once-a-year reviews and validations to ensure all case/utilization managers are well-versed or even aware of the topics related to status and hospital utilization.

Physician advisors need to keep abreast of all updates involving CMS rules and regulations and keep lines of communication open with the hospital contracting office to ensure they know about changes with payor policy. Any modifications in process (e.g., procedures removed from the Medicare Inpatient Only list) or additions of procedure (e.g., development of the Medicare Outpatient Observation Notice (MOON)) should be shared with the case/utilization managers promptly.

Hiring a Physician Advisor from the Ranks Versus from the Outside

As noted in the introduction, decades ago – when the payor landscape wasn't as convoluted as it is now, and the Two-Midnight Rule wasn't even a glimmer of regulatory innovation in some lawmaker's mind – physicians who became champions and experts in this field were generally well-established clinicians within the health system. They were widely known, well-respected, and integrated within the culture of the hospital. As such, they easily slid into conversations with other providers (especially older physicians, who commonly poo-pooed the new requirements and "impositions" placed on the medical staff) in an attempt to win hearts and minds.

However, this hyper-collegial approach carried a risk of backfiring. If the physician advisor was a 25-year golfing buddy with a surgeon whose documentation typically involved three lines of text, the message to "think in ink" might be delivered as an off-hand suggestion as opposed to a requirement for improvement. Likewise, if the physician was also responsible for serving as the vice president of medical affairs (VPMA), chief medical officer (CMO), or other time-consuming administrative position, addressing utilization and clinical documentation integrity (CDI) issues often fell to the bottom of the priority list. Chances might be slim that enough time would be allotted to addressing the needs of the case/utilization management team. As CMS rules involving Conditions of Participation (CoP) became more involved, it was no longer functional to have an individual addressing status reviews and utilization issues once or twice a week.

As the time pressures and scope of the role became more and more apparent, an increasing number of hospitals and health systems recognized the position of physician advisor required a singular focus and not simply be tacked onto another role's duties. But, finding established clinicians who were interested in moving into this administrative arena could be difficult. Many already were involved as VPMA, CMO, or medical director of clinical services in the inpatient or outpatient settings of the health system. For some hospitals which were able to identify individuals willing to take on the new position of physician advisor, they encountered many of the social and cultural challenges noted above.

These factors led some to expand their search for a physician advisor outside the walls of the health system. At first, the tactic may have been out of necessity without viable candidates within the confines of the system. Over time, advantages of bringing someone new into the fold became more apparent in some hospitals and developed into a required element. They found outsiders have no friendships or affiliations to protect when sharing frequently frustrating points of compliance and process improvement. They can be as blunt, straightforward, and strong-willed as needed along with projecting an element of humility, irreverence, and humor to interactions which could be hard to find in a long-standing, highly respected member of the established hospital community.

In-House Physician Advisors Versus "Hired Guns"

Almost as quickly as hospitals recognized there was a need for physician advisors, companies popped up providing contracted physician advisory services. Some health systems rely on these remote physician advisors for their status determinations across the board, but as time has gone on, more hospitals utilize this kind of service primarily when their employed physician advisor or advisors are off service.

An upside of using these remote physician advisory services is that they are always available when you need them. Nights, holidays, weekends…no problem. But, there are a number of issues which make this kind of service challenging as a hospital's primary source for physician advisors.

First, the CMS CoP state the Code 44 process (changing a patient covered by Fee-for-Service Medicare from inpatient status to outpatient status before discharge) must include an assessment by a provider on the hospital's Utilization Management Committee (UMC). In most instances, this committee is comprised of providers who are members of the Medical Staff Department. Since contracted physician advisors are not members of the medical staff, they are not on the UMC and technically cannot be the second provider involved in the Code 44 (the first being the attending provider for the patient).

Second, not being present within the hospital and unable to develop at least cursory face-to-face relationships with the providers makes it difficult to provide mentorship. If the providers are speaking with a different physician advisor over the phone each time a status question is raised, the lack of rapport could work against the provider taking the direction to heart. Instead, providers might settle into a position of simply agreeing with the status recommendation as opposed to truly incorporating the features of the case which support one status or the other.

A common arrangement, especially in hospitals where there is only one internal physician advisor, involves a mix of employed and contracted advisors. During the "work week," internal physician advisors are in-house; providing face-to-face education to their case/utilization managers and readily available to providers who are looking for clarification on challenging topics like custodial hospitalizations. Off hours, or, when the internal physician advisor is not present due to vacation or while attending a conference, routine status questions are sent to the remote service to address.

Advanced Collaboration Between Physician Advisors and Case/Utilization Managers

At the most basic level, case/utilization managers reach out to physician advisors when there is a question about patient status not addressed using MCG or InterQual guidelines. More advanced collaboration takes place when the physician advisor regularly provides education about commonly questioned scenarios, is receptive and enthusiastically encourages discussion about topics outside of status, and is involved in hospital departments outside of but connected to the sphere of CM.

Topics outside of routine inpatient versus outpatient status include the following:

1. Clues pointing to imminent or outright delays in patient care or discharge such as delayed procedures or imaging studies, specialty consult recommendations which are not acted on by the attending physician until the following day, or a patient's family member who is requesting discharge be delayed until the weekend.

2. Hospital utilization opportunities such as transitioning from intravenous to oral medications, pursing workups for conditions not requiring hospital care, or challenges with patient transportation home or to subsequent care facilities.

3. Appropriate status for patients presenting for planned surgical procedures, including pre-authorization by payors and identification of Medicare, Medicaid, or Tricare inpatient only procedures.

4. Custodial/social hospitalizations and how to identify them, along with targeted education not only for case/utilization managers but also providers, nursing staff, and social workers. This also dovetails into the appropriate use of the Advanced Beneficiary Notice (ABN) or Hospital-Issued Notices of Noncoverage (HINN) with patients covered by Fee-for-Service Medicare and in some cases, Medicare Advantage plans.

5. Collaboration between case/utilization managers and Clinical Documentation Specialists (CDSs) to identify opportunities in provider documentation which require more specificity and in turn, might lead to supporting escalation of patient status or supporting the patient's length of stay.

While it may appear to be a big leap for a hospital to hire their first physician advisor given the lack of a specific blueprint for the role, more and more are taking that leap and finding a myriad of benefits follow. Physician advisors consistently prove their worth and add value as physician champions to the CM Department, primary educator for the medical staff on "the business of medicine" as it relates to patient status, documentation integrity, and quality metrics. Physician advisors play a critical role within the system of opportunities involving anything from revenue cycle to the electronic health record and anything in-between.

Reference

American Academy of Physician Advisors (2020). Annual Member Survey.

Chapter 3:

Care Management Concepts

CONTINUUM OF CARE

Definition

The care continuum is defined as a system of care that guides a patient through various health services or different areas of healthcare over a period of time. This care continuum gives a path to the patient to navigate through the confusing world of healthcare. The role of the professional case manager (CM) is to help the patient effectively navigate through the continuum of care.

Successful navigation of the care continuum has been demonstrated to

- Improve patient health and safety
- Enhance the patient experience
- Avoid readmissions
- Control healthcare costs

The CM serves as the "hub," working with patients to safely and comfortably bring them from the hospital to home, through collaboration with the interdisciplinary care team across the internal and external facets of the care continuum. CMs accomplish this by educating and creating the crucial continuity necessary for patient success.

INTERNAL/EXTERNAL CARE CONTINUUM

The care continuum refers to the overall healthcare experience across multiple settings and provider types. It can be subdivided into "internal" and "external" categories.

Internal Care Continuum

In the acute care facility, the internal continuum is defined as the movement of the patient from presentation through discharge. Managing the patient efficiently and effectively through that time period and experience is important for CMs. Identifying delays in care, facilitating re-prioritization through collaborative communication, and asking key questions are all part of the daily management of the internal care continuum. *See Case Study 3.1.*

Case Study 3.1

During morning team huddle, the case manager is told the patient is being prepared for a colonoscopy that is scheduled for later that day. The case manager reviews the case, determines the colonoscopy is related to the reason the patient was admitted and is an appropriate procedure for the inpatient status. At the afternoon huddle, the staff nurse reports the patient has not yet had the procedure. The case manager calls the GI Lab and finds out the patient is not on their schedule for the day. In reviewing the medical record more thoroughly, the CM is unable to locate an order for the procedure. The CM calls the attending physician to get more information on the procedure and plan of care. This call reveals the physician had not ordered the procedure after a verbal consultation with the gastroenterologist two days prior. It appears that an overheard partial conversation was miscommunicated and then incorporated into the care plan without any team member verifying or validating the plan of care or order for the colonoscopy.

In "perfect case management world," the first step for the CM would be to verify and validate the presence of the order for the procedure, confirm the procedure was appropriate for inpatient status, and contact the GI Lab to ensure the patient was scheduled for that day. The CM follows the internal care continuum by keeping the patient informed of the anticipated time for the procedure, ensuring the completion of the procedure, and post-procedural documentation through collaborative communication. It's essential for the CM to eliminate delays and facilitate an excellent patient experience. The goal of case management is to facilitate efficient care, increased patient satisfaction, and lower costs of care for all.

External Care Continuum

The external care continuum refers to any linkage to care providers outside of the facility. The acute care facility is a small part of the healthcare continuum. Connecting the patient with external resources, providers and services is part of managing the external care continuum and helping our patients on the road to recovery and post-hospitalization success.

• Preventive Care/Screenings

• Family/Community Services

• Primary Care

- Specialty Care
- Pharmacy Services
- Behavioral Health
- Emergency Care
- Hospital Care
- Rehabilitation Services
- Home Health Care
- Long Term Care
- Non-Medical Home Care
- Long Term Community Supports/Services
- End of Life Care/Hospice/Palliative Care

See Case Study 3.2.

Case Study 3.2

"One day in late October, I received a call from a home health agency owner (Pete) regarding a patient referred to his home health agency from our in-house subacute rehabilitation unit (SAR). Mrs. K. was newly diagnosed diabetic who was admitted with a blood glucose >700. She had spent 3 days in acute care and 20 days on SAR to increase her level of function and had been discharged home with Home Health Services the day prior.

Pete reported that his team had been trying to get in contact with the primary care physician (PCP) prior to discharge to complete the process of confirming the PCP will be signing Home Health orders. He had received the initial referral on day 3 of her SAR stay. After multiple requests were sent, the PCP stated that she wants to see the patient first after discharge before signing home health orders.

Pete's team went out to the patient's home on the day after discharge per the hospital's physiatrist Home Health order to evaluate the patient. The patient reported that when she called to make follow up appointment with her PCP as instructed, she was told the next appointment available was in mid-December. The home health care team member also called to make the appointment for the patient, and they were told the same thing. Repeated calls yielded a possibility for an appointment in late-November, but no definite appointment could be given.

Pete called me and asked me to intervene, feeling the patient was at risk for readmission if care was not started ASAP and a follow up visit did not occur within the next few days. (Remember the gold standard for post hospitalization follow up is within 7 days of discharge.) I made a call to the practice manager, explained the situation and asked for an expedited appointment. They were unable to override their system and tried to put me through to the RN at the office; unfortunately, no answer. I left a voicemail. The representative sent an URGENT message and paged the MD directly to me.

I spoke with Pete again. We brainstormed on some ideas to get the patient connected with a temporary provider until her PCP could accommodate her appointment. I had attended a conference recently and had met a representative from a Home Visiting Physician service. I spoke to Claudia at the home visiting physician service and she stated that they would be able to see the patient and sign orders and care plan, pending the reconnection to PCP. I called Mrs. K., explained the situation, asked for her feedback and proposed the home visiting MD solution to her. She agreed to this.

In the meantime, I received a call from PCP who initially suggested the 4-6-week timeframe was acceptable, especially since she knew the patient so well. I asked if she was treating the patient for diabetes. She said that patient did not have a history of diabetes. I informed her of some of the details of her last admission, the new diagnosis of diabetes and her decreased functional capacity that required a stay in subacute rehabilitation. She stated she was unaware of these changes; despite the multiple attempts to communicate by the hospital and home health agency. The PCP indicated that she could facilitate a follow up visit in 14 days. I let her know that we had set up the visiting physician service to bridge between the current day and the appointment and she agreed with the plan.

The home visiting physicians took care of the patient until her appointment with her PCP and worked with home health care agency to facilitate her care and avoid an unnecessary readmission. Patient centered care, care coordination and collaboration! The strength of relationships in healthcare and the power of teamwork!"

(CMSA Chicago, 2019. C. Morley & E. Bergman, editors. Used with permission.)

COLLABORATIVE COMMUNICATION

Collaborative communication is essential in healthcare and is defined as "a higher level of joint working in which people and resources that may have previously operated in different spheres – separated by organizational and reporting relationships – are pooled together and aim towards a common end goal" (MyHub, 2019). This higher level of communication is the key to excellent patient management across the continuum of care. The primary drivers in this model are keeping the patient in the center of the discussion and respecting the input from all care team members. There are multiple effective formats for how team members can collaboratively communicate such as face to face huddles, daily rounds, conference, or video calls.

At its core, care coordination is just what the name implies: a mechanism through which teams of healthcare professionals work together to ensure that their patients' health needs are being met and the case manager is proactively advocating for the right care delivered in the right place, at the right time, and by the right person (Daniels, 2019).

Best Practices

- Collaborative Communication across the Interdisciplinary Care Team
- Look to internal as well as external continuum management
- Think outside the box for solutions to meet patient's individual needs
- Empower patients through education and connection with resources
- Connect with payer case manager to help break down barriers to transitions, authorizations and follow up.

References

CMSA Chicago. (2019). Case Management: It's Not Luck, It's Skill.

Daniels, S. (2019). Care coordination is not a synonym for discharge planning. RACMonitor, May 2019.

MyHub. (2019). Collaborative communication: Why it matters.

HEALTHCARE SURROGATE DECISION MAKERS

The CM recognizes that all individuals have a fundamental right to make decisions relating to their own medical treatment. Decision-making capacity is fluid and should be frequently assessed to ensure the patient can participate in the care plan decisions even when there is not a known living will or power of attorney for healthcare decisions.

The law that regulates decision-making in terms of individual personal decisions concerning medical treatment, lacks clarity and leads to uncertainty. It can be emotionally distressing for individuals involved in ethical decision-making without judicial involvement surrounding the right to self-determination. There are some circumstances where surrogate decision makers can make medical treatment decisions on behalf of patients without decisional capacity to terminate life-sustaining treatment, without judicial involvement.

Designation of Surrogate Decision Maker

When a patient lacks decisional capacity, the healthcare provider must make a reasonable inquiry as to the availability and authority of a health care agent under the Powers of Attorney for Health Care Law.

> A reasonable inquiry includes, but is not limited to, identifying a member of the patient's family or other healthcare agent by examining the patient's personal effects or medical records.
>
> If a family member or other healthcare agent is identified, an attempt to contact that person by telephone must be made as soon as possible after the provider determines the patient lacks decisional capacity.
>
> *Quoted from 755 ILCA 40/25; Illinois Healthcare Surrogate Law*

When no health care agent is authorized and available, the healthcare provider must make a reasonable inquiry as to the availability of possible surrogate decision makers. There may be laws defining this in your state and it is your responsibility to understand those laws.

Where there may be multiple surrogate decision makers (especially if prescribed by law), it is the responsibility of those potential surrogates to make reasonable efforts to reach a consensus as to their decision on behalf of the patient when choosing to forgo life-sustaining treatment. The CM can work with the surrogates during care conferences or goals of care meetings to establish consensus.

After a surrogate has been identified, the name, address, telephone number, and relationship to the patient are recorded in the patient's medical record. It is also a good idea to obtain a 'back-up" decision maker if the identified surrogate becomes unavailable or chooses to "step down" from the role.

The surrogate decision maker has the same right as the patient to receive medical information, medical records, and to consent to disclosure. This is not a HIPAA issue as the surrogate has a "need to know" status to make informed decisions regarding the patient's care.

Surrogate decision makers usually have the authority to make decisions for the patient until removed by the patient who no longer lacks decisional capacity, appointment of a guardian, or the patient's death. Again, it is important to know the laws governing your state in reference to this issue.

Utilizing guidelines that are available (state law or facility policy) for private decision-making will improve clarity to the process for implementing decisions concerning medical treatment and ultimately reduces the emotional distress for involved parties.

See Table 3.1 Comparison of Three States.

Comparison of Three States

Illinois	California	New York
Surrogate decision makers (per under 755 ILCS 40/ Health Care Surrogate Act) are listed as below in the following order of priority: 1. the patient's guardian of the person; 2. the patient's spouse; 3. any adult son or daughter of the patient; 4. either parent of the patient; 5. any adult brother or sister of the patient; 6. any adult grandchild of the patient; 7. a close friend of the patient; 8. the patient's guardian of the estate.	If a person lacks the capacity to make decisions, the physician and health care team will usually turn to the most appropriate decision-maker from close family or friends of the person. The most appropriate decision-maker is that person who has a close, caring relationship with the person, is aware of the person's values and beliefs, and is willing and able to make the needed decisions. This person may or may not be the person's next-of-kin. (This process for appointing a decision-maker has been common practice in California for many years though not in statute.)	Family Health Care Decisions Act (FHCDA) (Chapter 8 of the Laws of 2010, adding Public Health Law Ch. 29-CC and 29-CCC) Under the FHCDA, surrogate decision makers are listed as below in the following order of priority: 1. the patient's guardian of the person; 2. the patient's spouse; 3. any adult son or daughter of the patient; 4. either parent of the patient; 5. any adult brother or sister of the patient; 6. any adult grandchild of the patient; 7. a close friend of the patient.

Table 3.1 Comparison of Three States
Adapted from Illinois Healthcare Surrogate Act (2015), New York State Family Health Decisions Act (2010) & California Health Care Decision Law (2000). Table layout by author.

References

Illinois General Assembly: 755 ILCS 40/25. Healthcare Surrogate Act (2015).

NY Health Access New York State Family Health Decisions Act. (2010).

UCLA Health. (2000). California's Health Care Decision Law Fact Sheet.

PLAN/GOALS OF CARE MEETINGS AND THEIR PLACE IN CASE MANAGEMENT

Ellen P. Walker LCSW ACSW

Reason and Use of Plan/Goals of Care Meetings

Plan of care meetings in the past have focused either on illness such as end-stage renal disease, cancer or other life-threatening illnesses, or situations including rehabilitation. However, it can be argued the concept of the plan of care meetings can be extended to include end stage dementia patients and others (Murphy,et al, 2016). Since readmissions is a measurement of good care and hospitals have the responsibility of preventing these (Rennek, Nyguyen, Shoeb, and Magan, 2013.), a meeting that is centered around a patient's understandings of their illness, their goals of life, and medical options, may be a good place to begin.

Making your own healthcare decisions is something we take for granted today. The American Hospital Association Patient's Bill of Right includes "the patient has the right to make decisions about the plan of care prior to and during the course of treatment and to refuse a recommended treatment plan of care to the extent permitted by law and hospital policy and to be informed of the medical consequences of this action" (The American Hospital Association 2021). This was first adopted in 1973, and then revised in 1992. This ideal was also adopted by the Institute of Medicine in 2001, and by the American College of Physicians (Hernandez, Fornari, Rose, and Tortez, 2020). The Patient's Bill of Rights is still in continued use and reinforced by U.S. government standards and is considered a basic right for Medicare recipients (United States Publishing Office, 2018).

However, when this came out it was relatively a new concept. For decades, the physician and patient rested upon the notion that "the doctor knows best." Because of the adoption of the right to be involved in decision-making, plan of care meetings have been put in to use in many medical settings. You will find it in dialysis clinics, rehabilitation facilities, cancer clinics, and in hospitals; especially in situations involving palliative care choices. All of these areas share a common theme: to engage patients and their representatives in directing their own medical treatment.

The patient's values, ideas about quality of life, and how they want to live are essential topics of these meetings (Parrish, Kinderman, Rabow, 2015). The meetings will also review the patient's "medical history, current treatment, treatment options, prognosis with and without continued disease directed treatment and discussion with the patient's treating physician about the utility of the current treatment" (Parrish, Kinderman, Rabow, 2015). In other words, what is the patient's viewpoint of health and wellness? What is his/her past and current state of wellness? What could the future hold look like with or without treatment? These fundamental questions can only be answered by the patient and drive the entire interdisciplinary team focus.

The patient and/or representative(s) are also key to the meeting. The interdisciplinary team (IDT) is essential because it takes each team member's perspective to reach best outcomes for the patient. Members of the IDT include, physicians, nurses, case managers, therapists, nursing assistants, spiritual counselors, and social workers (Kefgen and Jones, 2015). Federal Certification standards for Long Term Care facilities also includes, food and nutrition staff and other appropriate professionals such as case managers and palliative care specialists. It is important to involve the patient in making decisions about their care.

The Goals and Structure of Goals of Care Meetings

The primary goal of these meetings is for the patient and their representatives to be heard and be an integrated part of the decision-making process. There are other focuses that come into play in the meeting. The following is cited by Parrish, Kinderman and Rabow:

1. Quality of Life—the opportunity for the patient and patient representative to provide information on how they want to live their lives. What does being alive mean to them?

2. Goals of Care—what are the patient's values and wishes and how does the IDT translate them into medical care goals for the patient?

3. Disease/Prognosis/Treatment options and its implications —come to an understanding of what the diagnoses and the treatment options are. In addition, what is the expected outcome of these options? These should be viewed from the medical, psychological, social, spiritual, cultural, and financial impacts on the patient's life.

4. Code status—now is the time to discuss patients code status. Do they understand what phrases like do not resuscitate (DNR) and full code mean? What is the patient's philosophy on these issues? Have they been documented?

5. Develop a holistic plan of care—where will the patient go from here? What direction will the plan of care take? What options for care will be employed and investigated? Make sure the plan encompasses the priorities of the patient and his/her representatives.

6. Advanced care planning—this is the time to discuss advance directives. Does the patient have a power of attorney for healthcare directive completed, or do they need one? Do they have a Physician Orders for Life-Sustaining Treat (POLST) met form? (2015)

All of these should be focuses of the meeting to make it successful for both the patent and the IDT. Focused goal setting prevents fragmentation of information and misinformation. It can also assist and support patients and their representatives in the healthcare decision-making process (Poojary, Levin, and Snyder, 2016).

There are two mnemonics often used to aid family meetings, **SPIKES** and **VALUE**. Both can are valuable in the actual running of the meeting, but also adds a tone of openness and inclusivity to the meeting. They have been developed to not only help the patient, but also to help the IDT.

The **SPIKES** model formulated by Buckmak is in six steps: (Baile, Buckman, Lenzi, Glber, Beale, & Kudela, 2000, reprinted 2021):

S—Set up the meeting Read the chart on the patient, research any possible options for care. Know your patient. Assemble the IDT. Prepare the patient and make sure the patient has support in significant others. Find a comfortable private area where there will be no interruptions.

P—Perceptions Find out what the patient and significant others perceive as the situation. What do they think is going on? What do they know about the patient's illness? What have they been told so far? Be sure to listen and pick up any inferred communication.

I—Invitation Invite them to tell you how they would like the information communicated to them. Do they just want to know the summaries of tests and examinations? Or do they want detailed information? Do they want to know specifics? Or a general overview? What do they want or need to know?

K—Knowledge Provide the information to the patient and support system, in a familiar and understandable way. Avoid using complicated medical terms, when possible. Speak in everyday language when able. Check for comprehension and understanding. Give information in small segments. Be careful to not overload them with too much information at one time. Use empathetic language to avoid startling bluntness.

E—Empathy/Emotions Listen and watch to observe how the patient and significant others may be reacting. Reflect what emotions you observe. If you have questions, be sure to ask them. How are you feeling? Check in with the patient and significant others regarding how they are experiencing the situation. Embrace moments of silence if needed. Give them time to process what has been said to them. Also, check into your own feelings. How are you reacting to the situation?

S—Summarize What are the possible outcomes for each option? What are the next steps? Will they actively treat the patient? Or is the plan to focus on comfort care? Is the patient returning home? What support is needed to get them there? Do they need to go to another facility for further care? How are the wants and the needs of the patient being balanced? What support systems and referrals need to be included? What is going to be the plan of care? Then summarize it to the patient and IDT. Make sure the patient and all parties involved are in agreement to the plan.

The other mnemonic is **VALUE** (Lautrette, et al, 2007), which was created to be more of a guideline to manage the interaction of the meeting than a step-by-step process but is none the less valuable.

The following are the ideals of VALUE:

V—Value family statements Be aware of what is being said. The family is impacted by the patient's decisions and their needs may be at odds. The patient and the family should have their values and needs heard.

A—Acknowledge Let them know you hear and understand them. Reflective listening is key in this situation. ("I understand you are concerned about...")

L—Listen Active listening is a skill which must be employed throughout the meeting. If you do not listen, you cannot value or acknowledge what the patient said.

U—Understanding Do you know what you are hearing? Is what was heard actually what is being said? Ask questions. Make sure you understand what the patient or other team members are saying. If you do not understand, chances are someone else doesn't either. Ask for further clarification.

E—Elicit Ask open-ended questions to ensure the patient and family understand the situation. Verify they know what is being said and try to bring to the surface any questions or concerns they may be holding back.

Both mnemonics are tools that can make plan of care meetings more successful. One is more pragmatic and the other more sensitive, but both put the patient at the center of the meeting and work with the patient's values, concerns, and needs to provide the care needed and wanted. *See Case Study 3.3.*

This study was a broad overview of what can occur in a plan of care meeting. Some meetings can be more general or work in small steps (taking one step at a time such as decisions on feeding tube insertion, resuscitation status dependent on family's coping skills) and some like above, will be more precise and detailed in choosing a complete path of care. Either way the meeting is geared to towards designing the patient's care around safety needs and wants of the patient or decision makers. In the above, the social worker and/or case manager plays several roles.

Case Managers and Plan of Care

In the scenario, the CM functions as a patient advocate. If Mary had verbalized any concerns herself, the CM may have reiterated Mary's feelings and wishes, advocating for the best solution to meet those patient centered goals. Also, the case managers and social workers are the gate keepers of services. They explain the support services available to patients and the financial aspects of their care. Their role is imperative to the team meeting as the discharge planning could not take place without it.

Case Study 3.3

Mary was an 83-year-old woman admitted to the hospital due to worsening dementia. Mary had lost her appetite and it was difficult for the family to get her to eat. She had been sleeping more and becoming less responsive to family. A swallow study showed no swallow deficits, but she continued to refuse food in the hospital and was becoming even less responsive. Mary was considered "full code" status, meaning all measures should be taken to save her life if needed.

A care planning meeting was called to discuss options for care. Since Mary was unable to speak for herself, her two daughters were asked to be present. Members of the IDT meeting included her hospitalist, speech therapist, a palliative care specialist, the chaplain, a dietician, and social worker and/or case manager. The family expressed feelings of frustration and concern. Despite their efforts to keep her actively engaged in life, Mary just seemed to continue to withdraw. The family asked if there was anything that could be done to help her.

The hospitalist explained that this was part of the process of severe dementia and although the medications she had been taking were able to slow the process, they could not cure her. He stated he did not see her condition improving. He suggested placing a feeding tube which may extend her life, but she would continue to worsen.

The speech therapist and the dietician also discussed the choice of continuing to feed Mary orally, letting her eat what and when she wanted. Palliative care discussed the option of comfort care measures and possible placement with hospice.

The social worker and/or case manager explained the services provided by hospice, along with supplemental homemaker services (to provide housekeeping, meal prep services), insurance benefits, and the Family Medical Leave Act (FMLA) that could help with providing the family more time at home with Mary.

The family was asked what Mary would have wanted. Her daughters talked about how active she had been and how much she loved her family, but that she probably would not have wanted a feeding tube. They were torn at thought of losing their mom, having lost their father just 18 months previously, but also felt they were just delaying the inevitable.

Spiritual support was provided to the family. In the end, the family chose to place Mary under hospice care and to change her code status to "do not resuscitate." The case manager referred them to a hospice agency and referred them to the state homemaker program. The case manager also assisted in advocating for the family with their employers to obtain the needed FMLA paperwork so they could be present to support their mother and each other through the dying process.

References

Allen, J., Hutchison, A., Brown, R., & Livingston, P. (2014). Quality Care Outcomes Following Transitional Care Interventions for Older People from Hospital to Home: A Systematic Review BMC Health Services 14, article number 346.

Apostol,C., Waldfogel, J., Pfoh, E., List, D., Billing, L., Nesbit, S., & Morss Dy, S., (2014). Association of Goals of Care Meetings for Hospitalized Cancer Patients at Risk for Critical Care with Patient Outcomes, Palliative Medicine. December 2014.

Baile, W., Buckman, R., Lenzi, R., Glober, G., Beale, E., & Kudelka, A. (2000, 2021), SPIKES–A Six Step Protocol for Delivering Bad News: Application to the Cancer Patient, The Oncologist, August 2000. Reprinted 2021.

Cook, D. & Rocker, G., (2014). Dying with Dignity in the Intensive Care Unit, *The New England Journal of Medicine*, June 2014

Hernandez, N., Fornari, A., Rose,S., & Tortez, L. (2020). Implementing Inter-professional patient-family centered plan of care meetings on an inpatient hospital unit. *Patient Experience Journal, 1*(11).

Jones, C., Hollis, R., Wahl, T., Oriel, B., Itani, K., Morris, M., & Hawn, M. (2016). Transitional care interventions and hospital readmissions in surgical populations: A systematic review. *The American Journal of Surgery, 212*(2), p 327-335.

Kefgen,L. & Jones, S. (2015). Patient Goal Oriented IDT Meetings: A Model to Identify, Plan, and meet Patient Goals, Across Hospice Disciplines.

Lautrette A, Darmon M, Megarbane B, et al. A communication strategy and brochure for relatives of patients dying in the ICU. *New England Journal of Medicine*, 356, 469–478.

Morley, C. & Walker, E. (2019). Health Literacy, Health Confidence and the Connection to Readmissions. CMSA Today, Issue 7, 2019.

Murphy, E., Froggatt, K., Sheelah, C., O'Shea, E., Sampson, E., Casey, D., & Devane, D. (2016) Palliative Care Interventions in Advanced Dementia, Cochrane Library Database of Systematic Reviews, December 2016.

Parrish, M., Kinderman, A., & Rabos, M., (2015). Weaving Palliative Care into Primary Care: A Guide for Community Health Centers, California Health Care Foundation, August 2015.

Poojary, I., Levin, C. & Snyder, L., (2016). Conducting Family Meetings, Elder Care A Resource for Interprofessional Providers, The University of Arizona, Arizona Center on Aging, March 2016.

Renke, S., Nguyen, O., Shoeb, M., Magan, Y. (2013). Hospital-Initiated Transitional Care Interventions as a Patient Safety Strategy, Annals of Internal Medicine, ACP Journals 2013.

United States Government (2018). Medicare and You 2018, U.S. Government Publishing Office 2018.

VanDonge, J., Wit, M., Smeets, H., Stoffers, E., Van Bokhoven, M., & Daniels, R. (2017). "They Are Talking About Me, But Not with Me": A Focus Group Study to Explore the Patient Perspective on Interprofessional Team Meetings in Primary Care.

Wolf, S., Berlinger, N., & Jennings, B. (2015). Forty years of work on end-of-life care---from patients' rights to systemic reform. *New England Journal of Medicine*, February 2015.

ADVANCE DIRECTIVES

Talking about or planning for end-of-life decision-making is a challenging topic that many people avoid having until it is too late. Who likes to think about this stuff? No one does. As professional case managers, we see the fallout of not thinking about this every day.

- Decisions having to be made during a time of crisis
- Families end up in disagreement about what to do for the patient
- Wrong person making decisions (estranged spouses or other family members)
- Some end up feeling like the "wrong decision" was made and would not have been what the patient would have wanted

Decisional Capacity: It's Not All or Nothing

Before turning to a Power of Attorney for Healthcare (POAHC) or surrogate decision maker, the patient must be assessed for decisional capacity. *(See Ethics: Decision Making Capacity on page 12.)* The patient may be able to make some decisions even if they can't make all of the decisions regarding their care. Patients who are minors should be offered the opportunity to participate in decision-making up to their level of understanding. Studies consistently show that decisions made by others are more aggressive and not as accurate as what the patient would choose.

Decision-Maker Priority

In the absence of a valid advance directive from the patient, there is an established hierarchy regulated by state laws to determine decision-maker priority. Check the state laws for the patient-specific surrogate decision maker algorithms. *See Healthcare Surrogate Decision Makers on page 77.*

Types of Advance Directives

- The professional case managers should be able to identify the different types of advance directives and their use. These are documents that state the patient's choices about medical treatment or name another person(s) to make decisions for their care if they can no longer make these decisions for themselves. Examples of these documents include:
- Durable Power of Attorney for HealthCare (POAHC)
- Living Will Declaration
- Do Not Resuscitate (DNR) Order
- Physician Orders for Life Sustaining Treatment (POLST)

Power of Attorney for Healthcare (POAHC)

POAHC is a legal document to designate another person(s) to make medical decisions for the patient should they become temporarily or permanently unable to make decisions for themselves. The POAHC can take effect at different points:

- immediately at the time of signing
- a future time elected by the patient
- when it is determined the patient can no longer make decisions on their own (this determination is decided by doctors providing care)
- can be revoked by patient with decisional capacity at anytime

The POAHC must be at least 18 years old and willing and able to perform the decision-making. This role provides the authority to:

- discuss the patient's condition, treatment plan, and options with the entire care team
- review medical records
- give consent for medical tests, medications, procedures and other treatments
- choose where care is received and the practitioners who provide care
- make end-of-life and final disposition decisions

Living Will

The living will informs the healthcare provider whether the patient wants death-delaying procedures given if they have a terminal condition and are unable to state their wishes at the time of care. The living will applies only if the patient has a terminal condition. A major stipulation in the living will is that food and water (nutrition and hydration) cannot be withdrawn if dehydration or starvation would be the primary cause of death.

DNR Form

Do-not-resuscitate order (DNR) is a medical order written by a doctor. It instructs healthcare providers to not perform cardiopulmonary resuscitation (CPR) if a patient's breathing or heart stops. A DNR allows the patient to choose whether or not they want CPR before an emergency occurs.

Do-not-intubate order (DNI) is a medical order written by a doctor. It instructs healthcare providers not to intubate and mechanically ventilate when a patient's breathing becomes difficult or stops. A DNI allows the patient to choose whether or not they want intubation before an emergency occurs.

POLST Form

In 1991, leading medical ethicists in Oregon discovered that patient preferences for end-of-life care were not consistently honored. Recognizing that advance directives were inadequate for patients with serious illness or frailty — who frequently require emergency medical care — a group of stakeholders developed a new tool for honoring patients' wishes for end-of-life treatment. After several years of evaluation, the program became known as Physician Orders for Life-Sustaining Treatment (POLST) (www.polst.org).

In September 2004 the National POLST Advisory Panel, later known as the National POLST Paradigm Task Force, convened to establish quality standards for POLST forms and programs and to assist states in developing POLST as a model process (or "paradigm"). The National POLST Paradigm Task Force was replaced with a new governance structure in 2017. POLST is now defined as a "portable medical order" (National POLST, 2020). Currently 32 states utilize the POLST form. To check on the adoption status of your state, access https://polst.org/wp-content/uploads/2021/07/2021.07.13-National-POLST-Form-Adoption-Map.pdf

The POLST includes provisions for living will and DNR status but does not include Healthcare Power of Attorney or Mental Health Treatment preference information. POLST is a process that allows patients to choose from a "menu" of all possible life-sustaining treatment, selected life-sustaining interventions, or comfort-focused care only. POLST is intended for persons of any age for whom death within the next year would not be unexpected, including patients with advanced illness or frail elderly patients. POLST is not intended for persons with chronic stable disability, who should not be mistaken for being at the end-of-life.

Use of the voluntary POLST promotes patient centered care by reducing the potential for errors by improving guidance during life-threatening emergencies. The form is designed to accompany the patient to any healthcare setting. As we know, in the absence of a POLST form, healthcare providers from first responders to physicians are required to offer all medically available treatment.

The POLST consists of three Primary Medical Order sections:

1. Section "A": Cardio-Pulmonary Resuscitation
Code Status – only when pulse AND breathing have stopped

Choices available:
- YES, perform CPR or
- NO, do not perform CPR

2. Section "B": Medical Interventions
Do Not Resuscitate does NOT mean Do Nothing

Three categories defining the intensity of treatment when the patient has requested DNR for full arrest but is still breathing or has a pulse.

- Full – all indicated treatments are acceptable
- Selective – no aggressive treatments such as mechanical ventilation
- Comfort-Focused – patient prefers symptom management and no transfer if possible

The patient and practitioner can elect to use the "Additional Orders" section for other treatments that might come into question (such as dialysis, surgery, chemotherapy, blood products, etc.). An indication that a patient is willing to **accept** full treatment should not be interpreted as forcing healthcare providers to offer or **provide** treatment that will not provide a reasonable clinical benefit to the patient (would be "futile").

Note that *Yes to CPR* in Section A requires full treatment in Section B. Why? If limited measures fail and the patient progresses to full arrest, the patient will be intubated anyway, thus defeating the purpose of marking *Comfort* or *Selective* interventions. However, selection of *Full Treatment* in Section B does not require CPR in Section A. Section B options are for Medical Emergencies aside from cardiac arrest. A person may wish to be intubated/mechanically ventilated in case of Respiratory Distress but would not want that treatment in the context of Cardiac Arrest. Section "A" choices influence medical interventions in Section "B".

3. Section "C": Medically Administered Nutrition

Medically administered nutrition can include temporary nasogastric (NG) tubes, total parenteral nutrition (TPN), or permanent placement feeding tubes such as percutaneous endoscopic gastrostomy tube (PEG) or jejunostomy tube (J-tube). A trial period may be appropriate before permanent placement, especially when the benefits of tube feeding are unknown, or when the patient is undergoing other types of treatment where nutritional support may be helpful.

4. Section "D": Documentation of Discussion

The form can be signed by:

- The patient
- The agent with a POAHC (when the patient does not have decisional capacity)
- The designated Healthcare Surrogate
    - when the patient does not have decisional capacity and has no POAHC or applicable Advance Directive
    - a parent of a minor child is a surrogate
    - a guardian is also a surrogate

The form must be signed by "one individual, 18 years of age or older, as witness to the signature of the patient or his/her legal representative's consent... A witness may include a family member, friend or health care worker" (National POLST, 2020). The witness CANNOT be the same practitioner as the one who signs the order. The CM may be asked to sign the form as a witness.

5. Section "E": Signature of Practitioner

The form can be signed by the primary care physician, attending physician, a licensed resident who has completed at least one year of training, a physician assistant, or an advanced practice nurse. If more than one person shares primary responsibility for the treatment and care of the patient, any of those persons may sign the order.

RECAP: Requirements for a Valid Form

- Patient name
- Resuscitation orders (Section "A")
- 3 Signatures
    - Consent by patient or legally recognized representative
    - Witness
    - Practitioner
- Date

All other information is optional for completion. The reverse side of the document has a section to notify if another Advance Directive is available, such as POAHC or Living Will. The National POLST organization recommends bright pink paper to enhance visibility, but the form color does not affect validity of form. Photocopies and fax copies ARE acceptable and legal.

Potential Concerns

- "The signing practitioner doesn't have privileges" at the facility the patient is currently admitted to.
    - Orders still must be translated into specific institutional orders
    - The National POLST organization suggests using "Pt is DNR per POLST form" as an order signed by assigned staff attending after review of the POLST form.
- "Our clinicians have never seen this patient before."
    - State laws indicate POLST orders must be honored in all care settings
    - Practitioners are protected from liability for following an POLST form in good faith
- Developing best practices for storing, locating, and transmitting documents between care settings

Case Study 3.4

Part 1

Ms. Jones is a 72-year-old female with Parkinson's disease who has been able to live at home and manage her own activities of daily living. A facilitated goals-of-care conversation is conducted by her primary care physician. Ms. Jones recognizes that her illness is terminal, and for that reason does not wish to undergo CPR in case of cardiac arrest. She has previously had discussed not being intubated with her family in the event of not being able to breathe on her own. She also vehemently refuses any consideration of feeding tube in the future. However, as long as her quality of life is good, she is willing to attempt less-invasive measures to prolong her life, as long as machine are not involved.

How should her POLST form be completed?

　　Section A: Do Not Attempt Resuscitation

　　Section B: Limited Additional Interventions

Part 2

Ms. Jones is admitted to the hospital with a urinary tract infection, significant weight loss and altered mental status. What life-sustaining treatments can be used? Should/could she be transferred to the ICU?

Because she said she is willing to attempt low-burden, less invasive measures to prolong her life, it would be reasonable to treat her with antibiotics and IV fluids. It is less clear whether she should have vasopressors or be transferred to the ICU if needed.

Part 3

She recovers and returns home. A month later, she is readmitted to the hospital with another urinary tract infection and continued weight loss. She is becoming more debilitated and requests to be considered for inpatient rehabilitation services to see if she can regain more function prior to returning home. She spends five days at an inpatient rehabilitation facility post-hospitalization and is unable to participate in rehab services. After a goals of care meeting, Ms. Jones decides to enroll in hospice services at home. Her quality of life has become acceptable to her, she no longer wants to spend time in the hospital and understands that her disease has progressed to a point where she will no longer be able to care for herself. More invasive medical procedures may be considered such as a feeding tube. Her POLST form should be updated to reflect these changes in Section B from Limited Additional Interventions to Comfort Measures Only.

Conclusion

Advance Directives conversations are hard conversations. They are also vital conversations. As patient advocates and champions of patient centered care, the CM is responsible for ensuring the patient has the opportunity to express their wishes for ongoing care should they be unable to communicate themselves. They also know the patient has the right to choose who makes decisions for them when they cannot. Ensuring that those conversations happen and serving as witness to the decisions made is well within the scope of the professional case manager's practice.

Chapter 4:

Transition Planning

TRANSITION/DISCHARGE PLANNING

OVERVIEW

Background and Goal

The transition or discharge planning component of acute care case management is a collaborative process of assessment, planning, facilitation, care coordination, evaluation, and advocacy for options and services to meet an individual's and family's comprehensive health needs through communication and available resources to promote quality cost-effective outcomes (CMSA, 2009).

According to the CMS Conditions of Participation, Discharge Planning chapter, acute facilities must have in effect a transition/discharge planning process that applies to all patients (2013). Transition/Discharge planning involves the appropriate post-hospital destination for a patient. The patient requires a smooth and safe transition from the acute facility to the next destination. This is the beginning of the process of meeting the patient's identified needs following discharge or transfer from the current facility.

> **Referencing the Transition/Discharge Planning Conditions of Participation from Medicare provides for a four-stage transition/discharge planning process:**
>
> - Screening all inpatients to determine which ones are at risk of adverse health consequences post-transition/discharge if they lack transition/discharge planning.
>
> - Evaluation of the post-discharge needs of inpatients identified in the initial screening or of inpatients who request an evaluation or whose physician/provider requests evaluation.
>
> - Development of a transition/discharge plan if indicated by the evaluation or at the request of the patient's physician/provider.
>
> - Initiation of the implementation of the transition/discharge plan prior to the transition/discharge of the patient.

Patient Rights & Responsibilities in Transition/Discharge Planning Process

CMS Conditions of Participation 42CFR 482.13 provides "the patient has the right to participate in the development and implementation of his/her plan of care and make informed decisions regarding their care" (2013). Patients or their representatives are actively involved in the transition/discharge planning process and the transition/discharge planner actively solicits information and input not only from patient or their representative, but also from family, friends, or support persons.

The patient should be afforded the right to participate in the development and implementation of his or her plan of care. The patient or representative (as allowed under state law) should be afforded the right to make informed decisions regarding care and be involved in care planning and treatment.

A patient has the right to refuse to participate in transition/discharge planning or to implement a transition/discharge plan. This refusal should be documented in the patient's medical record under Social Service interventions.

Transition/Discharge Planning Personnel

Transition/discharge planning evaluations must be developed by registered nurse, social worker or other appropriate qualified personnel or by a person who is supervised by such personnel (CMS, 2013).

Qualifications must include factors such as:

- previous experience in transition/discharge planning
- knowledge of clinical and social factors that can affect the patient's functional status at transition/discharge
- knowledge of community resources to meet post-transition/discharge clinical and social needs and assessment skills
- knowledge of clinical, social, insurance, financial and physical factors that must be considered when evaluating how a patient's expected post-transition/discharge care needs can be met

The process of transition/discharge planning should begin prior to or within 24 hours (or one business day) for all patients. The CM screens patients to assess their potential post-hospitalization needs. They work with attending physicians, social workers, patients, and families to assure continuity of care after transition/discharge. Screening and transition/discharge referrals also occur from other healthcare professionals such as nurses and ancillary services utilizing high-risk screening criteria.

INITIAL DISCHARGE PLANNING SCREENING AND ASSESSMENT

The CM assesses transition/discharge-planning needs within one working day of the patient's admission and initiates transition/discharge planning for nursing home or rehabilitation placement, durable medical equipment, home health care, hospice, transportation or other social supports/ services as needed (CMS, 2013).

Transition/discharge planning activities include provisions for, or referral to services required to improve or maintain health status following transition/discharge. Important factors considered for transition/discharge planning include, but are not limited to:

- Functional status
- Cognitive ability of the patient
- Biopsychosocial needs
- Patient's and caregiver's understanding of transition/discharge needs
- Identification of post-hospital care resources and family support
- Financial concerns (payer sources available, ability to pay for out-of-pocket services, limitations of potential coverages)

Professional case managers utilize screening tools developed for evaluation of self-care or alternatively, to be cared for by others in the environment or setting from which the patient was admitted prior to admission at the acute facility. In general, the goal upon transition/discharge is for the patient to be able to return to the setting in which they were living prior to admission. Assessment must include determination of whether patient is capable of addressing his/her self-care needs, resources available for care in the preferred post-acute destination, and services, medical equipment, and home modifications necessary for patient's successful transition.

If the patient, representative, support persons, or facility of origin are unable to address all of the required care needs, then the evaluation must determine the availability of community-based resources to meet the patient's needs while allowing the patient to remain in the setting of their choice. Healthcare services include, but are not limited to:

- Home health, attendant care, and other community-based services
- Hospice or palliative care
- Respiratory therapy
- Rehabilitation services (physical therapy (PT), occupational therapy (OT), speech therapy, etc.)
- End stage renal disease dialysis services
- Pharmaceuticals and related services
- Nutritional consultation, supplemental diets
- Medical equipment and related supplies
- Home and physical environment modifications
- Transportation services
- Meal services
- Household services, such as housekeeping, shopping, etc.

Results of the transition/discharge planning evaluation are required to be discussed with the patient/ representative and results of this communication are documented in the patient's medical record, including the patient/representative's acceptance or rejection of the plan.

Continued Stay Evaluation

During the patient's hospitalization, the case manager will reassess transition/discharge-planning needs as necessitated by changes in patient's condition or family's preference. Assisting those patients in need of additional resources includes, but is not limited to financial assistance, emotional support, counseling, and Medicaid and guardianship programs. All transition/discharge planning activities should be clearly documented in the patient's medical record.

Transfers to Another Acute Facility

In the event that a patient is transferred to another acute facility, any pertinent information concerning the identification of the patient's post-hospital needs should be in the patient's medical record that is transferred with the patient. The receiving acute facility then becomes responsible for continuing the transition/discharge planning process for the patient.

Patient Goals and Preferences

The acute facility should expect to engage the patient, or the patient's representative, actively in the development of the transition/discharge evaluation with the goal to incorporate the patient's goals and preferences as much as possible into the plan. Identification of unaligned hospital and patient assessments of post-acute expectations in a transition/discharge plan is imperative to facilitate discussion and resolution through development of a patient centered transition/ discharge plans that have a better chance of successful implementation.

TRANSITION/DISCHARGE PLAN IMPLEMENTATION

The acute facility is required to arrange for the initial implementation of the transition/discharge plan, including providing in-hospital education to the patient or caregivers for the care required in the home. Implementation also includes:

- transfers to rehabilitation hospitals, long term care hospitals, skilled nursing, or long-term care facilities
- referrals to home health or hospice agencies
- referral for follow up with physicians, providers, or outpatient services

- referral to medical equipment suppliers
- referral to pertinent community resources for assistance with finances, transportation, meal preparation, or other post transition/discharge needs

The patient/representative is required to be provided with information on:

- post transition/discharge options
- resources available for other non-medical post-discharge support (possible emergent provision of supplies, housing, transportation or food pantries, etc.)
- what to expect after transition/discharge and as applicable, instruction and training in:
    - how to provide care
    - what to do when concerns, issues or problems arise
    - who to call and when to seek emergency assistance
    - education regarding disease process, medications, treatments, diet, and nutrition

REFERRAL PROCESS FOR POST-ACUTE PROVIDERS OR TRANSFER TO OTHER ACUTE FACILITY

Referrals will be made for patients to transition to post-acute care providers (skilled nursing facilities, nursing facilities, home health agencies, hospice agencies, mental health agencies, dialysis centers, rehabilitation hospitals, long term care hospitals) or other short term acute hospitals to continue patient care. Additionally, referrals will be needed for suppliers of durable medical equipment, outpatient therapy providers, and physician offices to address needs identified in the transition/discharge planning evaluation.

Necessary medical information must be provided to the referral source to determine if the referral source can provide necessary care for the patient, has resources available at the time of referral, and meets the patient's and family's needs. Following HIPAA guidelines, the minimum necessary protected health information is to be used in making the referrals.

Medical information that could be supplied includes, but is not limited to:

- brief reason for hospitalization (history and physical or transition/discharge summary)
- brief description of hospital course of treatment
- condition at transition/discharge that includes cognitive functional status and social supports needed
- current medication list
- current allergy list

- current and pending laboratory work and test results
- current advanced directives, if applicable
- transition/discharge instructions, with follow up appointment identified

Referral information is sent to referral sources and the main contact for transition/discharge planning personnel with the decision. Acceptance or refusal by a referral source should be documented in the medical record and communicated to patient or representative. If more than one referral source accepts the patient for services, the patient or representative should make the choice of which option to pursue.

Best Practice

Communication of the transition/discharge plan and paperwork to the patient's primary care physician provides continuity of care along the continuum.

References

Center for Medicare and Medicaid Services. (2013). Conditions of participation for hospitals, discharge planning.

Resources

Conditions of Participation for Discharge Planning https://www.cms.gov/Regulations-and-Guidance/Legislation/CFCsAndCoPs/Hospitals

POST ACUTE LEVELS OF CARE/SERVICES

As mentioned throughout this book, I am honored to have the input and expertise of subject matter experts. This section is particularly illustrative of the expertise across the care continuum as each of the articles/topics covered in this section are written by experts practicing in that specific area.

SUBACUTE REHABILITATION UNIT (SAR)

Dr. Meghan Bisping DPT PT

Subacute rehabilitation (SAR) is a less intense level of inpatient rehabilitation services. SAR services are determined by the patient's condition and their ability to participate in ongoing therapy. Patients may be transitioned to SAR from the acute care facility directly or may transition from inpatient rehabilitation facility (IRF) to SAR as part of a step-down transitional plan. Patients can also transition from SAR to IRF once they have regained strength and tolerate longer therapy sessions. Transitions are assessed on a case-by-case basis.

SAR units can be located within acute care facilities or be in community settings such as skilled nursing facilities. Like those facilities, SAR units must be licensed by the Centers for Medicare and Medicaid (CMS) in order to provide SAR. They may also be accredited by the Center for Accreditation of Rehabilitation Facilities (CARF) to demonstrate excellence in care.

SAR facilities specialize in subacute care and provide targeted rehabilitation services. In SAR, the patient receives approximately one to two and a half hours of therapy each day, five to seven days per week with oversight from the medical team. Any changes in the patient's condition can be identified and addressed as needed.

As rehabilitation is the primary goal of SAR, the team of therapists—representing physical, occupational, and speech therapy disciplines—provide therapy to improve the patient's strength and functioning. This involves activities such as improving balance, safe ambulation practices, post-stroke recovery, and promoting independence with activities of daily living (ADLs).

Admission Criteria to SAR

- Patients need to demonstrate a functional decline from their previous level of function and be considered medically stable (stable weight and oral intake, afebrile).
- Patient cannot require 1:1 sitter
- Patient must be restraint-free for previous 24 hours prior to admission

- Patient must not be requiring any ongoing acute inpatient level of care
- Ongoing testing should be done as OUTPATIENT, even if the SAR is within an acute care facility. Tests such as cardiac catheterization, computed tomography (CT), magnetic resonance imaging (MRI), radiation therapy, surgical interventions, diagnostic x-Rays, and diagnostic laboratory tests will be scheduled as OUTPATIENT.

If progress continues steadily at rehab, the length of stay (LOS) is usually longer than in acute rehab. The LOS can be 14-21 days. The next step along the external care continuum for a SAR patient is usually at home with home health care, where a patient gets either home therapy and nursing visits, or outpatient rehab until rehab is finished.

The goal of SAR is to provide patients with time-limited services designed to improve functioning and to safely return the patient to their previous living environment. A variety of factors determine a patient's LOS at a SAR facility including:

- The extent of the patient's injuries or medical condition
- Patient's progress to goals
- Transition care for a safe discharge
- Approval for services by the patient's insurance carrier

SKILLED NURSING FACILITY (SNF)

Ericka Peterson MSW LCSW

Patients who are determined to have certain post-acute care needs, may benefit from admitting to a skilled nursing facility (SNF) at discharge. SNFs offer 24-hour nursing support for patients. This can be desirable for patients with certain medical needs who are concerned about meeting their care in the home environment. Patients also have access to physician care, medication administration, and skilled care provided dependent on their individual needs. During a patient's hospitalization, they are evaluated by different clinicians to determine their current and post-acute needs. SNFs can provide:

- intravenous (IV) antibiotics
- wound care
- peritoneal or hemodialysis
- physical therapy (PT), occupational therapy (OT), or speech therapy
- respiratory care
- nutritional support

It is common for patients to require antibiotics when discharging from the hospital. When patients require IV antibiotics, the care can be arranged with support from home health in the home environment or patients can choose to transition to a SNF. Patients often choose to go to a SNF for IV antibiotics because they may be more comfortable with the nurse administering the IV medication or may not have the support to administer the medication at home.

Patients with complex wound care needs may require SNF placement for post-acute care. If patients require daily wound care, are unable to manage their required wound care, or require specialized wound care (mist and ultrasound therapies), they may choose SNF placement. Although wound vacuum devices (wound vacs) can be arranged for use in the home environment, some patients prefer to admit to a SNF if they continue to need a wound vac at discharge. Dressing changes can also be done by medically trained staff in a SNF.

Patients are able to receive hemodialysis or peritoneal dialysis in a SNF. Some SNFs offer on-site hemodialysis which can be a convenient option for patients, rather than having to go off-site multiple times per week. It is less common for patients to receive peritoneal dialysis, but there are some SNFs that are able to accommodate this need and will often prepare their staff prior to the patient's arrival by performing specialized trainings to best support the patients through the process.

During a patient's hospitalization, they are often evaluated by PT and OT. These evaluations include post-acute recommendations, if applicable. Sometimes, they recommend patients admit to a SNF to receive subacute rehabilitation (SAR) which offers about one hour of PT and OT per day to patients while they are staying at a SNF. Patients may also be evaluated by a speech therapist to determine if therapy is necessary after leaving the hospital, and this can also be provided as part of SAR in SNF.

Patients may also receive respiratory care services while in a SNF. This can include oxygen administration, tracheostomy (trach) care, and ventilator support under certain circumstances. Patients who need to be suctioned more than once every four hours may require placement in a higher level of care than a SNF. There are limited SNFs that offer ventilator support for patients, which may also limit options for patients if they are ventilator dependent. If patients need to be weaned from a ventilator, they may benefit from admitting to a higher level of care, such as a long-term acute care hospital, which specializes in ventilator weaning.

Various types of nutritional support can also be provided in a SNF setting. This can include nutrition provided through a gastrostomy tube, jejunostomy tube, or a nasogastric tube (NG). Patients who present to a SNF with an NG tube, typically require a plan for discontinuation of the NG or a re-evaluation of their nutritional status. On rare occasions, patients can also receive total parental nutrition (TPN). Patients can also receive other dietary supplements dependent on their prescribed needs.

A patient's insurance coverage contributes to the type of care that is available to them. Patients usually have private insurance, Medicare, or Medicaid. Patients with private insurance plans choose facilities that are in-network with their insurance coverage. When patients have Medicare funding, they are eligible for SNF placement in most facilities. However, they are required to be in the hospital for three midnights prior to Medicare covering a SNF stay. They can stay up to 100 days fully covered for SNF needs. When patients have Medicaid only, this covers room and board at a SNF, but does not offer SAR. Patients with only Medicaid coverage are not able to get intensive PT, OT, or speech therapy in a SNF as Medicaid does not cover these services. Dependent on facility availability and policy, they may be able to reside custodially at the facility without any skilled needs.

When discussing the patient's post discharge plan, a list of facilities is presented to the patient based on facilities covered by their insurance, as well as by their geographic area of preference. If patients decide to proceed with SNF placement, referrals are sent based on their preference. Family members can also assist in the selection process if the patient wants. Three options are usually requested by a CM so that facility options can be explored simultaneously. Patients express preference for which facility they would like to pursue if they have multiple accepting facilities.

Once a patient has been clinically accepted by a facility, then the facility works on getting approval from their insurance. Authorization is required if a patient has a private insurance plan. This includes private Medicare plans, as well as private Medicaid plans. Clinical notes, physicians' progress notes, consults, lab work, medications, and evaluations are submitted to the insurance in order to get authorization for a patient to admit to a SNF.

When the doctors feel that a patient is medically ready to transition to a SNF, they alert the patient and social worker. The social worker reaches out to the facility to see if they have been able to obtain insurance approval (if applicable) and if they have available and appropriate space to accept the patient. Required isolation precautions are taken into consideration. Once a designated transfer time has been established, the patient's transportation is arranged based on the patient's needs. An ambulance is arranged if a patient is bed bound, oxygen dependent, requires isolation precautions, specialized monitoring, or positioning. If they are able to sit upright in a wheelchair, a Medicare is a more appropriate mode of transportation.

INPATIENT REHABILITATION FACILITY OR UNIT (IRF/IRU)

Jared "Jay" Johnson MSW LMSW CCM

There will be times that as a case manager (CM), there will be a patient who needs a form of physical rehabilitation. This could be physical therapy (PT), occupational therapy (OT), speech therapy (ST), recreational therapy (ROT), etc. Additionally, these patients might need to see a provider in an inpatient setting even though they are medically stable. Instead of keeping these patients in an acute care hospital setting, they may benefit from an inpatient rehabilitation facility, also known as IRF (or unit IRU).

IRFs are free standing hospitals, that primarily focus on intense rehabilitation for patients. A patient in one of these facilities must be able to handle three hours of therapy a day (CMS 2020). Additionally, these could be units that are attached to an acute care hospital. The IRF units that are attached to a hospital, are known as inpatient rehabilitation units (IRU). While the names are different, they operate under the same regulations, and have the same criteria levels for a patient to qualify for them.

How to qualify for an IRF/IRU

Skilled nursing facilities, long-term acute care hospitals, and swing beds, have inpatient requirements for admissions. IRF/IRU does not have an inpatient requirement. However, the patient needs to have a medically necessary diagnosis for admittance. Additionally, the patient will need to be able to handle three hours of intense therapy daily. Therefore, a patient could potentially present to an emergency room, or even a doctor's office and then be admitted to an IRF/IRU. However, most patients who are transferred to an IRF/IRU level of care, will do so after being treated for complex conditions.

The complex conditions, that would qualify include traumatic brain injuries, spinal cord injuries, cancer, organ transplants, major burns, complex trauma, strokes, and other neurological or orthopedic conditions (AHA, 2019). If the patient has Medicare for their payor source, then they must meet stringent criteria to ensure the level of care provided at an IRF is necessary. Additionally, if a patient has a Medicare advantage plan it is noteworthy that it is required to follow most of the Medicare guidelines, but advantage plans do not have to follow the same guidelines for IRF/IRU placement.

While it is not an ideal discharge disposition for the IRF/IRU (more on that later), it is worthy to note, that a patient who will need SNF placement, can meet their three midnights of inpatient while being at an IRF/IRU.

Differences between an IRF/IRU versus SNF

IRF/IRU provide a very specific service for patients. As a result, there are some major differences to be mindful of. Physician approval for readmission is required for IRF/IRU, while it is not required for a SNF. A patient who admitted at the IRF/IRU level of care will require resource-intensive inpatient care and will require close medical supervision by a physician with specialized training. Additionally, IRFs require the patient have physician coordinated multidisciplinary teams. CMS requires that nearly 80% of the discharges from IRF/IRU are to the community, while SNFs must have approximately 40%.

Case management working in an IRF/IRU

It goes without saying, that there are case managers (CMs) at the IRF/IRU level of care. While some aspects of case management at this level of care are different, there are many universal goals of case management. The most obvious goal is ensuring the patient is receiving the right level of care at the right time. Utilization management will also work differently at this level of care. While in an acute care setting the goal is the move the patient to the next level of care as soon as possible, that is not always the case with IRF/IRU settings.

Payment system for IRF/IRU

IRF/IRU receives a pre-determined payment for goods and services furnished during each Medicare recipient's stay in an IRF. The predetermined rates are based off of several factors including patient case mix and Medicare group IRF admitting condition. Patients admitted to this level of care are generally recovering from complex medical conditions. The level of need a patient has plus comorbidities and the admitting diagnosis, will indicate the Medicare approved length of stay (LOS) for a patient.

While the goal for an acute care setting is to move patients to the next level of care as quickly and safely as possible, that is not going to always be the case for an IRF/IRU. Patients will generally get approved for 10-20 days for IRF/IRU level of care with Medicare. Commercial insurances will approve or deny patients based off monitored progress. Prospective Payment System (PPS) coordinators will generally use the Medicare approved guidelines to determine LOS regarding payment. Every year CMS updates the rates to reflect inflation in furnishing IRF/IRU goods and services. Additionally, these rates are also intended to reflect changes in local wage rates.

Essentially, payment rates are determined by prospective payment systems. In addition to the admitting diagnosis, patients are further split into case mix groups (CMGs). The CMG is based off patients' level of need and comorbidities. For example, a patient who was recently treated for a complex stroke in the acute care setting, will generally get more pre-determined time in an IRF/IRU versus a patient who experienced an orthopedic trauma. Patients with more complex needs may have a higher risk of returning to an acute care setting or being discharged to a SNF, but the payments from Medicare will provide more payment based on the complexity of the patient. This is one of the many reasons why IRFs/IRUs have more scrutiny regarding compliance and outcomes.

Discharge Planning for IRF/IRU

The primary goal for discharge planning at the IRF/IRU level of care is to have safe discharges back to the community. Therefore, CMS requires that a certain percentage of discharges from IRF/IRU back to the community. The number of discharges that are required are reviewed annually. It is crucial that discharge planning begins upon admission. While in an acute care setting, not all patients will require the assistance of a CM or a discharge planner, it is highly probable that each patient will require assistance with discharge planning at the IRF/IRU level of care.

While CMs will have to have some discharges to a SNF/NH, these locations are not the primary goal. It's important to note, discharges to a personal care home or assisted living will count as a community discharge. Therefore, CMs may need to work on securing acceptance for an assisted living facility or personal care home. The actual act of completing a referral to an agency is not any different than many other levels of care. If a patient can meet the requirements of the assisted living facility or personal care home and has the financial means, then it is encouraged to seek placement at an assisted living facility or personal care home. Discharges to inpatient hospice will not count as a discharge to another institution.

While the IRF/IRU, does require physician approval for admitting to the facility, there are times that a patient will be admitted to the IRF/IRU, and in fact are not able to handle the intense therapy or have a need for that level of care. Typically, the attending following the patient will notify the CM if this is the case. When a CM is notified of this scenario, it is important the CM work on moving the patient to the appropriate level of care. Sometimes this may be a SNF or nursing home (NH) placement. CMS does allow for a percentage of patients to be discharged to that level of care. If the attending physician does not feel the patient is at the appropriate level of care, the CM for that patient will be tasked with finding the correct level of care in a timely fashion.

Additionally, it is not uncommon for CMs at the IRF/IRU level of care to be responsible for managing follow up appointments. Any time a patient must go to a doctor's appointment, the IRF/IRU facility must pay for that appointment. Furthermore, when a patient is not available for therapy, that is less therapy the patient will be able to do. At the same time, some appointments may be medically necessary such as a follow up appointment with a surgeon for an orthopedic trauma patient. Appointments with the patient's primary care doctor are not considered medically necessary. Patients are being followed closely by an attending in the IRF/IRU. Any needs the patient has from their primary care doctor can be managed by the attending.

A CM at this level of care could face potential conflicts for discharge planning. Some of these will include unrealistic expectations. For example, a patient who has a percutaneous endoscopic gastrostomy (PEG) tube and will likely need it for an indefinite time, and their family may not feel comfortable with how to use the PEG tube for feedings. However, CMs can arrange for the family and patient to be educated on how to care for and use a PEG for feedings and providing medications. This will not only set the patient up for success, but it will also avoid transitioning the patient to a SNF/NH level of care. Additionally, families can be educated by the therapist regarding the level of assistance a patient may need at discharge. This education provides the family members the required education to give safe assistance they are caring for the patient after discharge. Overall, the CM may be responsible for coordinating education for patients and families regarding the needs of the patient after discharge.

Of course, case management is not ALWAYS rainbows and sunshine. CMs will have cases that do not fall into ideal situations. This is where you, will use the basic concepts of best practices and apply them to a case. The logistics of how each IRF/IRU operates on a day-to-day basis will vary. However, this section is intended to provide a basic concept for IRF/IRU.

LONG TERM ACUTE CARE HOSPITAL (LTCH)

Erin Cunningham BSN RN CCM

Long term care hospitals (LTCH) are certified as an acute care hospital. They are required to meet the same Medicare Conditions of Participation (CoPs) as acute care hospitals paid under the Inpatient Prospective Payment System (IPPS). To meet the Medicare designation of LTCH eligibility for the Medicare Severity-Long Term Care-Diagnosis Related Groups (MS-LTC-DRGs) assigned at discharge, the hospital is required to maintain a Medicare average length of stay (ALOS) greater than 25 days.

The inpatient hospital stay at a LTCH are reimbursed for discharges under the LTCH PPS. The MS-LTC-DRGs are the same Medicare Severity Diagnosis-Related Groups (MS-DRGs) that CMS uses under the IPPS. LTACH MS-DRG Payment System is unique because it is calculated to hospital-specific base rates, based on historical discharge data, each DRG assigned a relative weight, and DRG assigned ALOS.

Criteria

The enactment of the 2013 Bipartisan Budget Act (Public Law 113-67) provided clinical criteria for admitting to LTCH beginning for cost reporting periods beginning on or after October 1, 2015. Section 1206(a) of Public Law 113–67 amended section 1886(m) of the Act to establish two criteria points for admission.

First, the patient admitted directly from an IPPS hospital with at least three days in an intensive care unit (ICU) or coronary care unit (CCU) but the discharge must not have a principal diagnosis in the LTCH of a psychiatric or rehabilitation diagnosis. The second clinical criteria, the patient have been admitted directly from an IPPS hospital and the LTCH discharge is assigned to an MS-LTC-DRG based on the receipt of ventilator services of at least 96 hours, but must not have a principal psychiatric or rehabilitation diagnosis in the LTCH.

The regulations at CFR 412.522 specifies that immediately preceding discharge is from a "subsection (d) hospital." This means that a hospital located in one of the 50 states or the District of

Columbia—other than certain specified IPPS-excluded hospitals such as, LTCHs and psychiatric, rehabilitation, children's, and cancer hospitals (see §412.503). The patient may have had an immediately preceding inpatient stay at a subsection (d) hospital that is not present in the Medicare claims processing system. An example of this scenario would be a military treatment facility utilizing their Veteran Affairs benefits facility that qualifies as an "immediately preceding" stay. LTCH will need to submit clinical documentation with claim to demonstrate clinical criteria met to avoid Site Neutral payment.

Section 1206(a) of Public Law 113–67 amended section 1886(m) of the Bipartisan Budget Act to establish patient-level criteria for payments under the LTCH PPS for implementation beginning for cost reporting periods beginning on or after October 1, 2015. The patient-level criteria creates two payment categories known as Site Neutral and Standard payments.

The "site neutral" amount will be paid for patients discharged from the LTCH that do not meet one or both above criteria. Any site neutral paid case will be excluded from the calculation requirement for LOS.

Best Practice

Communication of the transition/discharge plan and paperwork to the patient's primary care physician provides continuity of care along the continuum.

References

Centers for Medicare and Medicaid. (2018). Long term care hospital services.

Centers for Medicare and Medicaid. (2020). Long term care hospital prospective payment system. Medicare Learning Network, MLN Matters, March 2020.

HOME HEALTH CARE

Peter Miska RT

It seems the 20% rule applies to most things in life. In healthcare, 20% of the patients consume 80% of the resources. These patients are the highest risk for hospitalization or being considered superusers of healthcare resources. These patients must be identified, and case managed with diligence. The characteristics of these patients according to claims data from the Centers for Medicare and Medicaid, are as follows:

- Age 75 or older
- Three or more active health conditions
- Two or more falls in the last three months
- Low health literacy
- Functional deficits requiring PT and or OT
- Five or more prescribed medications
- Inadequate support system
- Incontinence
- Shortness of breath
- History of non-compliance
- Two or more hospitalizations in the last 12 months
- Weight loss, reported self-exhaustion, slower movements sit to stand and while walking
- Cognitive impairment and or recent decline in mental/ emotional or behavioral status
- Dementia (2019)

Home health agencies can keep these patients out of the hospital by providing patient education, protocols, office-based care coordination, and case management. Patients and caregivers are educated about diagnoses. Clinicians follow several comprehensive disease specific protocols, including chronic obstructive pulmonary disease (COPD), diabetes, heart failure, pneumonia, joint replacements, etc. Targeted education involving the patient and caregiver is designed to increase adherence to the plan of care and prevent further hospitalization. The use of telehealth and case management will become the industry standard. CMs will make daily contact with the patient and caregivers to assess the health status of patients.

In response to any abnormal findings, the CM will contact the patient to triage the situation. If warranted, a same day visit will be performed. The physician will then be notified to prevent an ER visit and subsequent admission to the hospital. Early prevention and detection are the key in this process. To succeed, home health agencies must be proactive in addressing prevention, utilization, compliance, quality, outcomes, spending, and patient satisfaction.

Medicare Home Health

To qualify for the Medicare home health benefits the Centers for Medicare and Medicaid have established the following criteria:

- The patients must be confined to home (homebound)
- Be under the care of the physician
- Be receiving services under a plan of care established and periodically reviewed by a physician
- Require skilled nursing care on an intermittent basis, physical therapy, speech-language pathology therapy, or have a continuing need for occupational therapy
- Need a face-to-face encounter with an allowed provider type as mandated by the Affordable Care Act (2019).

The homebound criteria per Centers for Medicare and Medicaid (2019), include:

For Criteria One, the patient must either:

- Have an illness or injury where the patient needs supportive devices such as crutches, canes, wheelchairs, walkers, the use of special transportation, or the assistance of another person to leave their place of residence

OR

- Have a condition that leaving his or her home is medically contraindicated.

If the patient meets one of the Criteria One conditions, then the patient must also meet the two additional requirements defined in Criteria Two.

Criteria Two includes:

- There must exist a normal inability to leave home and leaving home must require a considerable and taxing effort.

In order for a home health agency to accept a patient, they will require:

- A patient's demographic sheet listing name, address, phone number, and insurance information.
- A written order for home health care services from a physician and/or allowed provider type i.e., RN/PT to evaluate and treat because/for: diagnosis and reason for home health services.
- Recent physician visit note, progress note, or discharge summary including a patient's history and physical and a current medication list. This is referred to as a "face to face" encounter or simply, a "face to face". The concept is that home health care services are being ordered by a provider who has met with, visualized the patient's current functional status and ongoing medical needs and is attesting to the patient's need for this level of service.
- A home health Certification Statement, signed, credentialed, and dated by the MD or allowed provider type (date used on Certification Statement for face-to-face encounter must be the same date as the visit/progress note provided to the agency).

Review Choice Demonstration

The review choice demonstration (RCD) for home health went into effect in Illinois on June 1st 2019. Florida, Texas, Ohio, and North Carolina will be the next states enacting Review Choice Demonstration (RCD). RCD is the response to fraud concerns from the Medicare Payment Advisory Council (MED PAC), Office of the Inspector General (OIG), and General Accounting Office (GAO) because, on audit review, improper payments for home health care services were determined to be 17.2% in 2013 and 59% in 2015. A Pre-Claim review demonstration program was implemented for 26 weeks in 2016-2017 in Illinois alone, that identified over $100 million in savings surrounding fraud investigations and agency closures.

With RCD, the Medicare Administrative Contractor or MAC will conduct the reviews. This will not create new documentation requirements for the home health agencies. The services will begin in a timely fashion. Home health agencies would have three options for their review choices including:

- Pre-claim review
- Post-payment review
- Minimal post-payment review with a 25% payment reduction

If pre-claim review is chosen, it is required for each episode including re-certifications. If affirmed a Unique Tracking Number (UTN) is assigned for final claim to bill. If it is not affirmed, the agency can correct the problems or documentation and submit as many times as it takes to make it right. This is the case if they do not bill a final claim without the UTN. These requests may be submitted by fax, mail, or electronically submitted to the MAC and the initial UTN turnaround time is one to ten days.

The focus of RCDs is:

- Medical necessities
- Homebound status
- Being under the care of the physician
- A plan of care established and periodically reviewed by a physician
- Must have or need intermittent skilled services.

Documents supporting payment and coding rules are:

- Referral documents
- Comprehensive Outcome and Assessment Information Set (OASIS) form
    - (OASIS is the patient specific, standardized assessment tool used in HHC to create care plans)
- Accurate ICD-10 coding

- A plan of care signed by an MD or allowed provider type
- A face-to-face encounter
- Any clinician notes and the verbal orders.

Payment Model Changes

On January 1, 2020, the Patient Driven Grouping Model (PDGM) was implemented to replace the Prospective Payment System (PPS) reimbursement. PDGM does not rely on the number of therapy visits performed to influence payment. Instead, it relies on the principal diagnosis, functional level (low, medium, or high from the OASIS assessment), admissions source (community or institutional), comorbid conditions (from the patient's secondary diagnosis), and the 12 clinical groupings (such as neurology, rehabilitation, wounds, etc.).

The grouping model uses 30-day billing periods of care in a 60-day episode. Approximately 60% of 60-day payments are paid in the first 30 days, and 40% of 60-day payments are paid during the second 30 days. Institutional referrals are patients that had an inpatient stay from a hospital, Skilled Nursing Facility (SNF), Long Term Care Hospital (LTCH), or Inpatient Rehab Facility (IRF). Community referrals are patients without a documented inpatient stay. Community referrals will be paid at an approximate 20% discount of an institutional referral. Observation stays and emergency room referrals from the hospital without an inpatient stay are considered community referrals. There are 432 different payment categories in PDGM.

About 40% of the diagnoses that were allowed under the PPS will not be accepted as primary diagnosis under PDGM. Questionable encounter codes are "too vague," meaning the code did not provide adequate information to support the need for home health services. Under PDGM, claims for "questionable encounters" will be sent back to the agency as "return to provider" (RTP), since CMS will not be able to assign the 30-day period to one of the 12 PDGM clinical groups.

For example, "code is too vague and not specific enough (Muscle weakness, generalized M62.81). A better code would be a more diagnosis specific such as G20.0 for Parkinson's disease, G35.0 for Multiple Sclerosis, or R53.81 Deconditioning and general debility.

What Home Health Diagnoses Will No Longer Be Covered?

Here are the most used home health diagnoses that Medicare will no longer cover after 2020 for Home Health Care:

> **ICD M62.81:** Muscle weakness (generalized)
>
> **ICD Z91.81:** History of falling
>
> **ICD R26.89:** Other abnormalities of gait and mobility

ICD R26.81: Unsteadiness on feet

ICD R29.6: Repeated falls

ICD R53.1: Weakness

ICD R29.6: Unspecified abnormalities of gait

ICD R26.2: Difficulty in walking, not elsewhere classified

ICD S72.001D: Fracture of unspecified part of neck of right femur, subsequent encounter for closed fracture with routine healing

ICD S72.002D: Fracture of unspecified part of neck of left femur, subsequent encounter for closed fracture with routine healing

ICD S81.801D: Unspecified open wound, right lower leg, subsequent encounter

ICD S81.802D: Unspecified open wound, left lower leg, subsequent encounter

ICD I13.2: Hypertensive heart and chronic kidney disease with heart failure and with stage 5 chronic kidney disease, or end stage renal disease

ICD I12.0: Hypertensive chronic kidney disease with stage 5 chronic kidney disease or end stage renal disease

ICD M19.90: Primary osteoarthritis, unspecified site

ICD M19.90: Unspecified osteoarthritis, unspecified site

ICD M06.9: Rheumatoid arthritis, unspecified

ICD C34.90: Malignant neoplasm of unspecified part of unspecified bronchus or lung

ICD Z46.6: Encounter for fitting and adjustment of urinary device

ICD R33.9: Retention of urine, unspecified (Centers for Medicare and Medicaid, 2019)

The Impact Act was implemented into law on September 28, 2019. One of the goals of the act was to standardize the information collected between the four post-acute care providers (PAC). This includes the functional, cognitive, special services, treatment, intervention, medical conditions, co-morbidities, and impairments. The PAC providers are SNFs, IRFs, LTCHs, and home health agencies (HHA). Hospitals must provide the patient with a list of HHAs to choose from. Then, the hospitals must follow the patient's choice and document it in the medical record. Patients want facilities to have five star ratings, low hospitalization rates, determined value, and positive patient experiences. *See The Impact of the IMPACT Act of 2014 on page 235.*

Bundled Payments after hospitalization for PAC providers are becoming the new norm. Low cost care, high-quality services, and patient satisfaction are the measures. Located below is an episode window for a 90-day Home Health bundle after an inpatient stay. HHAs will be measured on all part A/B spending for the 90-day period. *See Bundled payments for care improvement on page 241.*

Since 2016, home health value based purchasing (HHVBP) has been in effect in nine states (Arizona, Florida, Iowa, Maryland, Massachusetts, Nebraska, North Carolina, Tennessee, and Washington) and will be expanded in January 2022. In the HHVBP program, the lowest performing agencies will receive a pay reduction. The highest performing ones will receive pay increases for several measures (+/- 8%) based on the agency's ability to improve patient outcomes. High star ratings will be imperative for an agency's success. Located below are a few of the indicators that are being measured (Center for Medicare and Medicaid, 2019).

Table 4.1 shows the star ratings of the 11,802 agencies in the United States (January 2019). Five- and four-star agencies will receive pay increases in HHVBP, 3-star agencies will be neutral, and 2.5 stars or less will receive payment reductions (Centers for Medicare and Medicaid, 2019).

5 Stars	512 Agencies (4%)
4.5 Stars	997 Agencies (8.4%)
4 Stars	1,324 Agencies (11.3%)
3.5 Stars	1,611 Agencies (13.8%)
3 Stars	1,586 Agencies (13.4%)
2.5 Stars	1,260 Agencies (10.8%)
2 Stars	964 Agencies (8.2%)
1.5 Stars	377 Agencies (3.2%)
1 Star	43 Agencies (0.4%)
No Stars	3,128 Agencies (26.5%)

Table 4.1 Star Ratings of the 11,802 Agencies in the United States.

From Centers for Medicare and Medicaid, 2019. Table layout by author.

References

1800HOMECARE. (2019). New payment system would reject nearly one in five home health claims. Will access to care continue?

Centers for Medicare and Medicaid. (2018). Home health services.

Centers for Medicare and Medicaid. (2019). Patient driven payment model.

Centers for Medicare and Medicaid. (2020). Home health patient-driven grouping model.

Graham, J. (2020). Why home health care is suddenly harder to come by for Medicare patients.

Resources

Home health services. https://www.medicare.gov/coverage/home-health-services

Patient driven payment model. https://www.cms.gov/Medicare/Medicare-Fee-for-Service-Payment/SNFPPS/PDPM#fact

HOSPICE CARE

Metoda Posega RN CMSRN

What Is Hospice Care?

Hospice care is a specialty program and philosophy of care that focuses on person at the end of his or her life rather than treating the disease. Hospice care is offered to patients with advanced illness. It could be cancer, end stage heart disease, end stage dementia, or someone who suffered a stroke. The disease must be severe enough that there is no aggressive treatment option.

Criteria

Age does not matter and will not qualify or disqualify a patient for hospice care. Two physicians have to qualify patient for hospice care. The physician refers a patient to a hospice care agency when it is believed the patient does not have any aggressive treatment options or they would prefer comfort care treatment. The physician's professional opinion is the patient has less than six months to live if no aggressive treatments were pursued.

Hospice treats physical pain as well as emotional and spiritual distress. Hospice does not hasten someone's death. The hospice program consists of highly skilled registered nurses, home health aides, social workers, and volunteers who specialize in end-of-life care and are able to support patients and families in different settings. Some hospice agencies also have board certified music therapists. Hospice is not a place, however hospice can be provided in a nursing home setting, short stay in a hospital setting, or at an inpatient center. Most of the time the hospice care is provided in patient's home where the staff will visit.

Hospice is covered by Medicare part A at 100%, as well as by Medicaid and other insurances. Durable medical equipment is also covered under hospice benefits (hospital bed, oxygen, wheelchair, commode, etc.). Some medications are covered to treat pain, agitation, and shortness of breath. Hospice provides different levels of care:

- routine level of care at home where the patient is comfortable and has good family support
- general inpatient level of care
- respite care
- continuous care
- bereavement for 13 months after death

Hospice does not provide care givers to stay with patients. Some hospice companies have their own specialized inpatients centers that a hospice patient can be admitted for short term treatment of symptoms (pain, agitation, shortness of breath) or for five days of respite to give the family a break as caregiving can be exhausting.

Admitting Process

Primary care physicians or specialists can determine the need for hospice care. If a patient has been deemed unable to make their own decisions or elects to have another person act as decision-maker, the physician will contact the family member who is the decision-maker and will discuss hospice care. Once the patient or decision-maker agrees to hospice care, the order will be placed, and the CM will further discuss hospice services and available agencies to choose from. A referral packet is sent to the chosen agency and once accepted, the chosen agency will reach out to patient or decision-maker. Then an appointment will be scheduled to meet with a hospice representative. At the hospice meeting, goals of care will be discussed, questions are answered, and the hospice election benefit form and consent are signed. At this time, the Physician Orders for Life Sustaining Treatment (POLST) form may also be signed. The POLST form is not a requirement for obtaining hospice services. *See Advance Directives on page 87.*

HOME CARE

Aishling Dalton Kelly CADDCT CFRDT CMDCP

Home care is exactly as the title suggests: it is the delivery of care in the home for wherever one calls home. Home care can be delivered in the actual home setting of the patient or client. It can also be delivered in a community type setting such as a memory care, assisted living, or an independent care facility. Home care offers two lines of services, hourly (shift work) or live in (continuous care for a daily rate) where caregivers live in the home setting. When choosing the live in option, the home care agency abides by labor laws for sleep and meal times for the caregiver on site.

Home care is emerging as a frontrunner and is frequently requested because research demonstrates that people experience better outcomes in the security of their own home when recuperating post-operatively or from an illness. Non-medical home care delivers assistance with activities of daily living. Some examples of these activities are personal care needs for bathing and showering, medication reminders, daily exercise, laundry, meal preparation, errands, socialization, activities, and transportation to doctor appointments.

How Is Home Care Paid For?

There are very few ways to pay home care. One of the biggest misconceptions is that Medicare pays for home care—but this is not the case. Often, home care and home health get confused. Home health is paid for by Medicare, however, home care is not. One of the ways that home care can be paid for is if the patient or client has a long-term care insurance plan. If so, the home care company and/or the recipient of the care can submit the paperwork. The client is reimbursed following the delivery of services.

There are also veteran programs available. Qualified veterans can receive a specific number of hours weekly under the veteran plan of care. Home care agencies must be contracted with the Veteran's Administration (VA) to take care of these type of clients. In addition, there is a veteran assistance program where veterans can receive a stipend for additional hours of assistance.

Clients or patients may be able to get home care under the state's Medicaid program. Again, certain conditions apply, and this is typically for patients within lower income brackets. The last way to pay for home care is called private pay, which means the care is paid for out of pocket.

How Does a Referral Get Submitted?

All home care agencies must be licensed under the Department of Public Health (DPH). Under this licensure, all home care companies must be insured, bonded, pay all taxes for their employees, fingerprint, background check, and continually educate their employees. A complete list of licensed agencies is on each state's DPH website. This list should be updated annually, and cross checked against the previous years' lists for validity.

Best Practices

- Get to know the health care associations and professional organizations in your area such as the Home Care Association of America. These organizations can be helpful to gain a referral of a reputable agency.
- Case Management Society of America has members from the home care arena.
- The Seniors Blue Book Discharge Planner Resource Guide is a great referral assistant that lists the home care agencies, their areas of coverage, and services offered.
- Internet searches are another way to find agencies. It is highly-recommended to speak to a minimum of three agencies before selecting an agency without a professional referral.

Case managers working in hospitals should become familiar with local home care agencies to establish safe and reliable pathways for discharging patients requiring homecare. One of the best way to learn about referral resources is to build relationships and network with other healthcare professionals by attending educational events and joining professional associations.

DURABLE MEDICAL EQUIPMENT (DME)

Wendy Jaffe MSN RN CCM

One of the most important components of a patient's discharge is arranging durable medical equipment (DME) for the patient to transition to the home setting. This will ensure a safe discharge for the patient to return home and will often prevent a readmission. DME consists of various assistive devices that will help the patient achieve the most independent environment in their home.

Prior to the patient's discharge to home, an assessment should be made by the therapy department to determine what equipment is needed. This assessment can be done by a physical or occupational therapist. Their expertise is vital in the discharge planning process for the patient to become as independent as possible in their homes.

Once the assessment is completed, the therapists will then consult with all the healthcare providers involved in the care of the patient. The case manager (CM) or discharge planner uses the recommendations made by the therapists to provide an all-encompassing discharge plan.

The next step is to determine what kinds of DME the patient needs. Depending on the piece of equipment needed, the physician will document in the medical record the medical necessity for the equipment. This is extremely important for the equipment to be covered by the patient's individual insurance plan. If the patient has traditional Medicare, there are strict guidelines to follow for documentation of medical necessity for that piece of equipment. The CM educates the physician on what is needed to justify the DME. Each insurance plan will cover the equipment needed once the medical necessity is documented and approved by the plan. Each individual piece of equipment has criteria that must be met to be approved. There may be co-pays for the equipment needed. When there is a co-pay, it is explained to the patients to make them aware of their individual cost.

The CM uses the equipment company that is considered in-network with a patient's private insurance plan or managed Medicare or Medicaid plans. If the patient has Medicare or Medicaid, then any company may be used that can provide the equipment that is recommended.

Depending on what is needed for the patient, the equipment can be delivered to the patient's room prior to discharge or to the patient's home. There are some companies that require the patient to pick up the equipment at their warehouse—which would require an additional conversation with the patient. Make sure you communicate the process for obtaining the equipment clearly to the patient and family, so they know what is expected.

DME can be several different kinds of devices such as:
- Oxygen therapy
- Wound care supplies (wound vac)
- Bathroom equipment (commodes, transfer benches, and shower chairs)
- Mobility devices (walkers, wheelchairs, and rollator walkers)
- Enteral supplies that are used if a patient cannot eat but has a gastric tube, nasal gastric tube, or total parenteral nutrition (TPN/PPN)
- Any other equipment the therapist decides is important in maintaining independence at home

The essential DME that is obtained for the patient provides a safe and optimal home setting for the patient to transition into.

TRANSITION/DISCHARGE PLANNING TOOLS

Our "toolbox" is important. This next section helps to identify tools, resources and gives perspective and tips from a front line case manager on best practices.

STANDARDIZED REFERRAL PACKET

West Suburban Medical Center Case Management Department, Oak Park, IL

Transition plans can change on a day-to-day basis. Best practices for transition planning include the use of post-acute services to make multiple referrals simultaneously across the continuum. I often say "a good case manager has a plan A, and plan B all the way through Q if needed."

To facilitate this process in a timely manner, West Suburban Medical Center in Oak Park, Illinois, worked with their post-acute provider representatives for their Continuity of Care Network to create a universal standardized referral packet for all levels of post-acute care. The rational for standardization was to decrease the time spent in creating individual referral packets This process was made even easier once electronic medical records were implemented.

Process

The following will be included in all referrals to outside agencies, home health, hospice, skilled nursing facilities, acute rehab centers, and long-term acute care hospitals.

- Face sheet (demographics)
- Order or transfer sheet
- Discharge instructions
- Medication administration record (MAR) or any medications from the discharge instructions
- History and physical
- Home medical equipment ordered and the DME company's name and phone number
- For home health patients, a "face to face" physician assessment encounter documented for those with Medicare *See Home Health Care on page 111.*
- Last two to three days of physician's progress notes
- Up to date lab values (including hepatitis panels, toxicology)
- Physical, occupation, or speech therapy evaluations and progress notes from the last three days
- Copies of consults
- Current vitals

- Dialysis times and dates (if applicable)
- Social work discharge planning notes (make sure contact numbers are correct)
- Name and number of primary physician, or name and number of resident physician who will be following and his/her preceptor's name and number. If a patient is unable to leave the home for a clinic appointment, please request a home visiting physician. If a patient is going to a nursing home, include the name and number of the attending physician on the case, including hospitalists.
- Department on aging and rehabilitation services referral (if applicable)

For patients with additional specialized needs, additional information may be included in packet as needed.

COMMUNITY RESOURCES: VALUABLE TOOLS FOR CASE MANAGERS

Janet Coulter MSN MS RN CCM

According to pocketsense.com, community resources are the businesses, public service institutions, and charitable organizations that provide assistance and services to local residents. A community resource is anything that has the potential to improve the quality of life in a community, defined by the Community Tool Box (University of Kansas, 2019).

The traditional definition of community resources includes organizations, support groups, and outreach groups that focus on helping people. A broader definition includes public services such as the library, churches, and business that serve the community, as well as individuals who work to improve community life by helping others. Community resources can help meet certain needs and improve the quality of life for the individual, family, and community. These resources can be managed or funded by the government, businesses, non-profit groups, or even individuals, and serve the community in a variety of ways.

Although many community resources remain unused due lack of awareness that they exist or uncertainty about how to access them. Case managers (CM) utilize community resources every day. These resources can be used to provide for client's basic needs (food, clean water, clothing, shelter, and medical care) and to assist clients with financial, housing, and medication needs.

It is important for CMs to be aware of resources available in their communities. Although a complete list of community resources is not possible and is ever changing, this section will provide suggestions for accessing community resources.

Community Resources

The Centers for Disease Control and Prevention (CDC) report "working at the community level promotes healthy living, helps prevent chronic diseases and brings the greatest health benefits to the greatest number of people in need" (Centers for Disease Control and Prevention, 2018). The wide range of community resources can touch the lives of everyone in the community. Resources may include community health organizations, as well as services specific for individuals or smaller segments of the community. These resources are valuable to assist, maintain and improve health, prevent the spread of infectious diseases, and prepare for natural disasters.

When searching for community resources, be sure to identify what type of assistance is needed to narrow the search. Frequently used community resources include:

- County human services: food stamps and Medicaid assistance
- Food banks: food for anyone who cannot afford to buy groceries
- Private charitable organizations who can help pay utility bills one time
- Hospitals, clinics, and public health organizations: assistance for those who do not have private insurance coverage or financial resources to see a healthcare provider. Many providers offer a sliding scale fee based on income that allows uninsured or underinsured clients to access health care services. Others have charity care applications available for this population. Check with your institution for specific information.
- Churches, synagogues, ethnic leagues, and veterans' associations.
- Public schools: free or reduced-price meal programs for students during the summer and during breaks, adult continuing education, tutoring, books, literacy and GED preparation classes, English language acquisition classes, and access to computers for free or at the lowest cost possible.
- The Head Start Program: services to both parents and children from low-income families. These services include education, health, and nutrition services.
- Red Cross: resources to shelter community members during weather-related emergencies.
- The March of Dimes: assist families with neonatal or pediatric healthcare.
- There are several community resources that offer assistance to young adults on issues such as pregnancy, substance abuse, suicide prevention, and educational counseling.
- Community resources to assist the elderly population.

Conclusion

There are many community resources available for CMs. Our role as CMs is to identify and meet our client's comprehensive health needs. This includes linking clients to available community resources. Some clients need more assistance than others, and there is no shame in seeking out additional resources to optimally support the patient. While there were several resources listed, it is not a comprehensive list of community resources. It may take some investigating to find the appropriate resources, but that research and passion to help our clients is what helps define us as professional CMs.

References

Centers for Disease Control and Prevention. (2018). NCCDPHP: Community Health.

Kentucky University (2019). Section 8: Identifying Community Assets and resources.

Staff Writer (2020). What Is the Meaning of Community Resources?

University of Kansas (2019). Community Tool Box.

Resources

theanswerhub.com provides information for the elderly in a specific community

www.justfindinfo.com provides information for Senior assistance

www.samaritanspurse.org provides assistance for families and children

https://www.cdc.gov/tobacco/stateandcommunity state and community resources regarding smoking and tobacco use

United Way's 211 Information and Referral System dial 2-1-1 or text the zip code to 898-211 for referrals to utilities and food pantries

https://www.unitedway.org supports programs for health, education and financial stability

https://www.rd.usda.gov provides financial assistance programs for a variety of rural issues including housing

www.suicidepreventionservices.org provides suicide prevention information

https://grantushope.org mental wellness, safety and suicide prevention in schools

https://cmsa.org Case Management Society of America

https://www.nursingworld.org American Nurses Association

https://www.acmaweb.org American Case Management Association

Pharmaceutical companies: many can provide prescription medications free or at a reduced price

Pharmacy discount programs like GoodRx, Inside RX

Local pharmacy discount programs: offered at CVS, Walgreens, Walmart for example

Department on Aging – state specific/provides adult protective services and services for adults with disabilities

Diagnosis Specific Sites: https://csn.cancer.org, https://liverfoundation.org, https://diabetes.org and other national organizations may be able to provide financial support for specific disorders. www.lupusresources.com provides a co-pay program that helps eligible patients

https://www.cdc.gov provides resources and recommendations to prevent chronic diseases and promote health across the life span https://www.medicare.gov provides information about Medicare coverage

https://victimconnect.org/resources/national-hotlines/ provides a 24-hour support line

Workers Compensation: contact state office for information and then ask for a case manager

Community websites: provides information about community resources and names of people who may be of assistance

Town directories

Bulletin boards

Friends and colleagues

Local Senior Citizen organizations and Senior Centers

Community clothes closets: provide clothing free or at a reduced price

Local community mental health centers treat and provide support for individuals with behavioral health disorders

COMMUNITY RESOURCES: NOT A NATIVE TO THE COMMUNITY, NO PROBLEM!

Mariana Turgeon MSN RN CCM BSCS

I had moved from Northern Virginia where I had lived for over 20 years, to the more rural Richmond area. For six years I gained familiarity with the area by using Google Maps, but was concerned when I transitioned into case management because I was not as familiar with community resources needed to properly transition children from the inpatient acute hospital settings to their homes.

Learn About Your Area and What's Available

The first thing I did was to work side by side with the other pediatric intensive care unit (PICU) CM to obtain a "simple" copy of their resource list. This resource list was the most valuable source of information to get me started. It was a great start but the days of three-inch case management binders are long gone. Utilizing the multiple electronic resources to keep track of resources is imperative. Password keepers, spreadsheet software, and electronic phone lists allowing quick access to resources are key to helping connect our patients with resources.

The second most valuable piece of advice is to obtain a notebook and write everything down. Either a spiral notebook, composition notebook, business day planner, steno notebook, or even an expensive hard back journal that you can carry around everywhere you go. Write down everything, even tiny notes! Make sure you date the pages because it can be daunting to look through the notebook for that primary care provider you spoke with that made it a mission to take care of medically complex children.

I found the charge nurses had a lot information too. One of the charge nurses was local to the Richmond area and I noticed many of her co-workers looked up to her because she was a wonderful teacher and preceptor to the new nurses in the unit. Many of these PICU nurses have since become Nurse Navigators in the specialty or community pediatric offices. They enriched my networking with the community. They were able to rely on me when they needed discharge planning help for their patients in their community offices because I had established a strong rapport.

It's essential to figure out which companies you can rely on to gather supplies for patients. It is our job as CMs to offer choices and fortunately, in adult healthcare there are many choices. Unfortunately, in the pediatric world, there are not as many choices. There are minimal home health and DME companies that provide care for pediatrics. The DME or home health orders need to be specific to reduce ambiguity.

Research

Google can be a wonderful tool for locating resources by using specific key words in searches (food pantry, homeless shelter, domestic violence shelters, etc.). Google can be an excellent resource for locating those "one-off" requests. Local "Areas on Aging" offices, state public health departments, or human resources websites can be great starting points as well. The example below is from the Illinois Department of Human Services website. Other resources can be subscription services such as Healthify, Aunt Bertha's, FindHelp.

Use an Electronic Fax Cover Sheet

If a referral for home health must be manually faxed, make sure a fax cover sheet precedes the order. The cover sheet should not be handwritten, but filled out electronically with a text editor like Microsoft Word. Use a fax form template and annotate your contact information – name, phone number, email (at the minimum) and most importantly make sure the patient's name and date of birth is on the fax form. Electronically save a copy of the fax form so that you will have the resource contact information the next time. The recipient will also have your contact information in case there are any issues with the order. It takes valuable time to hand write a fax cover sheet which can lead to mistakes when transferring the information. As you save each form, you eventually have more contacts that are used sporadically. In addition, utilizing an electronic fax form looks much more professional than a handwritten form that is hard to read.

Ask the Questions!

I believe one of the most important community resources are the patients and their families. They are the ones out in the community navigating the social services system. Listen to their experiences, make note of resources they may be using for future reference that could be useful for other patients. Do not be afraid to ask questions about social determinants of health and community resources they access to fill those gaps. (See Special Topics on page 197.)

Take Discharged Patient Calls!

Many times, the families need help with "paperwork" like obtaining new orders, Family Medical Leave Act (FMLA), or just a note showing they were at the bedside with the patient during the admission. Do a deep dive and find out if you are the best person to help the caller. Do not be afraid to look into the chart to see which case manager helped them during their inpatient stay. Maybe they know more about this patient than you. Make sure to annotate in the chart why you accessed the patient information so that there is no misinterpretation later why your name was logged into a chart you had not performed case management services. Do NOT pass the call to someone else UNLESS you know that person can provide the help they need. I can attest that those families REMEMBER the help (good and bad). To provide excellent follow up care, case managers should have business cards to give to their patients for any post-discharge questions.

Social Networking

Stay abreast of resources that can help you in your job. Join reputable case management social media groups that support your mission. Groups moderated by professional organizations or well-known thought leaders in case management are the best choices. Many barriers that you identify have probably already been put out there by other case managers. Networking is a key to uncovering those hidden gems of community resources. Do not be afraid to state a general request for resource assistance. Do not include any patient or situation specific information. You will reap the benefit of multiple CMs' experience in one place.

Resources

Healthify, formerly Purple Binder https://www.healthify.us/

Aunt Bertha's FindHelp https://www.findhelp.org

TRANSITIONS AND CARE COORDINATION PERSPECTIVES

The acute care case manager does not work on an island. True care coordination involves hand-overs across the care continuum. This section brings together transitioning from acute care to other care settings and the perspectives of those next level of care case manager partners. Working together is key to a patient's success. It is valuable to the acute care case manager to understand how those partner case manager's impact transitions.

POST ACUTE CARE COORDINATION / PCP

Anne Albitre LMSW CCM

Hospital readmissions are costly and often avoidable. Successful care transitions from the hospital to the community reduces fragmentation in healthcare and readmission risk. "Each year, roughly 2 million patients are readmitted, costing Medicare $27 billion, of which $17 billion is spent on readmissions that could be classified as potentially avoidable" (Kaufman, 2016). Studies suggest primary care providers (PCPs) report a lack of communication from inpatient to outpatient care, communication not performed in a timely manner, and necessary information is missing or unclear. The World Health Organization, The Joint Commission, and the Australian Commission on Quality and Safety in Health Care identify care transitions as a cause of preventable morbidity (Johnson et al., 2012).

> **The Joint Commission (2016) lists these factors that may increase risk of readmission:**
> - Diagnoses associated with high readmissions
> - Co-morbidities
> - The need for numerous medications
> - A history of readmissions
> - Psychosocial and emotional factors, such as issues relating to mental health, interpersonal relationships, or family matters
> - The lack of a family member, friend or other caregiver who could provide support or assist with care
> - Older age
> - Lack of transportation or funds to get medications post-discharge

While barriers to smooth transitions of care cannot always be fully eliminated, there are several best practices that can be used to facilitate care transitions from acute care settings into the community. Centers for Medicare and Medicaid (CMS) uses the term "transitions of care" to describe transferring a patient from one care setting to another (Mansukhani, 2015). For example, a transition of care could be from an acute care hospital to the patient's home with home health services. Care coordination from the acute care setting to community providers, and across the continuum of care is extremely important. Failures to follow best practices can lead to negative outcomes for patients, increased readmission rates, and disruptions to the patient's healthcare recovery.

Mansukhani et al (2015) identifies evidence-based strategies for improving provider communication and reducing readmissions which include: effective provider communication, using health information technology, medication reconciliation, ensuring access to care after discharge, communication of healthcare information, and follow-up telephone calls.

Other best practices when transitioning a patient from acute care into the community include assessing patients at each admission, following up on referrals to ensure there are not gaps in care, scheduling outpatient appointments before discharge, and ensuring patients have the resources and knowledge needed to make informed choices for quality care.

Key Strategies Checklist

- ☐ Effective Provider Communication
- ☐ Use of Health Information Technology
- ☐ Medication Reconciliation
- ☐ Access to Care Post-Discharge
- ☐ Communication of Healthcare Information to Patients/Caregivers
- ☐ Follow Up Post Discharge
- ☐ Providing Quality Choices of Services

Effective Communication and Using Health Information Technology

A meta-analysis by Kripalani et al. (2007) found direct communication from hospitals to PCPs occurred at a rate of only 3-20%. The research also demonstrated 66-88% of the time, discharge summaries were not available to outpatient providers at the time of post discharge and were missing significant information such as discharge medications, follow up plan, diagnostic test results, and treatment or hospital course.

Centers for Medicare and Medicaid (CMS) recommend providers issue a summary of care for all transitions of care or referrals. Public Health and Promoting Interoperability Programs (formerly Meaningful Use) is a CMS program that sets specific objectives that eligible professionals (EPs) and hospitals must achieve to qualify for Medicare and Medicaid Electronic Health Records (EHR) Incentive Programs. One of these objectives is the Electronic Exchanges of Summary of Care. This objective state that EPs who transition their patients to another setting of care or provider of care, or refer their patient to another provider of care, should provide a summary care record for each transition of care or referral (Gillingham, 2020, p.106).

Medication Reconciliation

"The Agency for Healthcare Research and Quality (AHRQ) describes the problems in care transitions as 'systematic' and the cause of most adverse events arise after discharge. Lack of effective communication between inpatient and outpatient providers is a significant contributor to medication safety errors upon discharge" (TJC, 2016). Medication reconciliation should be completed at every transitional point of care. The goal is to provide correct medications to patients at every point of care. Errors, discrepancies, contraindication, and omissions have been linked to rehospitalization and studies show that 46-56% of all medication errors happen during care transitions (Mansukhani et al., 2015).

The Joint Commission (2016) states:

"safe, quality transitions of care can serve as safety nets for accurate medication management and good quality outcomes for patients. Each transition of care is an opportunity to ensure better patient safety across the continuum of care, starting at admission to a health care facility, throughout the visit or stay, at discharge, and following through to the next care setting."

Ensuring Access to Care After Discharge

Mansukhani et al (2015) recognizes ensuring patient access to care after discharge as an important role in ensuring smooth care transition. This includes ensuring patients have access to DME such as home oxygen therapy, mobility assistive devices, and medications. Some hospitals provide bedside medication delivery, while many pharmacies will now deliver medication right to your home. Prevent gaps in care post discharge by assessing and navigating patient barriers to obtaining care after discharge such as lack of transportation to the pharmacy, prior authorization requirements, cost of medications, or co-pays. This may help initially, but referrals to social work or community resources may help resolve long term problems impacting access to care.

Communication of Healthcare Information

Communication of healthcare information to patients and families can be impacted by health literacy. Gillingham (2020) defines health literacy as "the ability to obtain, communicate, process, and understand basic health information." Gillingham (2020) goes on to say that nearly 9 out of 10 adults in the United States do not have proficient health literacy and are not proficient in understanding health-related information. More than one third of adults in the United States have difficulty following directions on their prescription label. Communication of healthcare information to patients can also be limited due to disabilities in hearing and vision or cognition impairments (Mansukhani et al., 2015).

Studies show that patients understand and retain about half of the information given to them by providers and they often do not feel comfortable asking questions or asking providers to repeat information. As a case manager, you should speak slowly, use plain language, avoid medical jargon, reinforce key information, provide printed and visual instruction materials that are easy to read, and use the teach back method by asking questions like "please tell me in your own words what we have discussed" or "what would you tell your family about your condition?" (Cornett, 2009).

Referrals for tests, consults with other providers, treatments, or procedures can be a problem for individuals with low health literacy. Often the patient is told to read the referral form and call to make an appointment. The patient in this situation has to find out where to go, follow instructions given to prepare for the referral, determine if insurance will pay for the service, and complete a new registration form or additional paperwork. All of these steps can be an overwhelming task for anyone, but especially for those with low health literacy skills.

The referral process can be made easier by helping patients in the following ways (Mayer & Villaire, 2007; Weiss, 2007):

- Make written instructions clear and simple, using language that is easy to read and understand.
- Review the instructions with patients and check to be sure they understand the information.
- If procedures require preparation, ask patients to tell you in their own words what preparation is required.
- Place directions to the referral site and/or a map on the back of the referral form and review the directions with them.
- Help patients with insurance issues. Call for an appointment for the patient before they leave the facility (Cornett, 2009).

See *Special Topics: Health Literacy on page 206.*

Follow Up Post Discharge

Follow up telephone calls to patients post discharge improves patient care transitions. Calls 24 to 72 hours after discharge can address immediate patient needs. Hospitals who have implemented follow up telephone calls to patients have focused on discharge medication list, barriers obtaining medications, and patient health issues (Mansukhani et al., 2019).

Providing Quality Choices

Sometimes when patients who live independently in the community are recommended to discharge to a skilled nursing facility (SNF), they decline this type of placement. Many patients who decline placement have had negative past experiences with SNF or nursing homes, and instead desire to return to the community with home health services. Almost inevitably, they are readmitted.

A study by Tyler et al., (2017) looked at the post-acute care placement process and found case managers simply gave a list of agencies to patients and did not attempt to inform them of which agencies were of better quality. They interviewed 138 staff members and all but 1 reported giving patients a list of SNFs with no qualitative information. The study found staff members believed patient choice regulations prevented them from providing information about facility quality. Most patients selected the closest SNF to their residence. When asked if they would travel further if a higher quality of care SNF was recommended to them, 75 of the 98 patients said they would have.

> "While it is true that Social Security statutes guarantee Medicare patients the right to choose their providers, nothing in these statutes precludes hospitals from helping patients make an informed choice. In fact, while CMS interpretive guidelines say that patients should be provided with a list of facilities near their homes, the guidelines also say that discharge planners may direct patients to the quality data available on the Nursing Home Compare website" (Tyler et al., 2017, p. 1390).

Assisting patients and their families in choosing high quality care settings and navigating resources to make informed decisions can support a more successful discharge plan that leads to better patient outcomes.

The IMPACT Act of 2014, enacted in September 2019 requires hospitals to empower patients in their care transitions "and improves quality by requiring hospitals to provide patients access to information about post-acute (PAS) provider choices, including performance on important quality measures and resource-use measures" (CMS, 2019). A patient who receives care at a higher quality facility is more likely to have better outcomes, less likely to experience readmission and more likely to return to a facility in the future if medically necessary. Case managers should be proactive in staying up to date on regulations and recommendations from CMS and other regulating or accrediting bodies. *See Special Topics: The Impact of the IMPACT Act of 2014 on page 235.*

A Day in the Life of a LMSW

As a Licensed Medical Social Worker (LMSW) case manager for a primary care doctor clinic, I provide transitions of care for our Medicaid and Medicare patients who have been hospitalized. My patients are typically high utilizers and are considered high risk for readmission. Most of my patients discharge back to the community, but some require SNF or nursing home placement. In my position, I have access to real time health technology informing me when our patients are admitted. When the patient is admitted, I make contact with their hospital case manager for care coordination, schedule a post hospital PCP appointment, and provide appropriate information to the hospital case manager on the patient's social situation, specialists and barriers to care or adherence. I contact the patient telephonically within 24-48 hours post discharge and provide case management services for up to 30 days in order to reduce chances of readmission.

When I identify one of my patients is admitted, I attempt to make contact with their hospital case manager right away, especially if there has been a significant change since their last admission. "Communication across an interdisciplinary team, including the doctors, nurses, pharmacists, insurers, skilled nursing properties, home health agencies, and others involved in the care of the resident, may result in reduced risk of readmission, and therefore keep overall costs down" (Kaufman, 2016). Many times, other providers involved in the care of the patient will have information you do not have or information the patient does not give you, even after completing an assessment with the patient. Confirm the information you have is the most up to date information.

Once the hospital case manager communicates an estimated discharge date, I coordinate to schedule a PCP appointment for within seven days of discharge. A study by Tong, et al. in 2018 found that a patient was more likely to have a follow up visit if it was scheduled prior to their hospital discharge at 30% compared to less than 5%. A visit within two days post discharge had the greatest reduction in readmission rate and visits after two days were still significant, but less significant over time.

When patients need to follow up with outpatient providers, some hospital case managers will schedule the appointment for them. If feasible, schedule outpatient follow up appointments prior to the patient discharge, place it in their discharge summary and instructions. When appropriate, educate the patient, caregivers and family on the importance of attending the appointment and the reason for the appointment. Assess for barriers to attending and adjust as needed. Communicating with outpatient providers about patient admission and scheduling follow up appointments will help facilitate a warm handoff and you can use this opportunity to obtain needed information to issue a summary of care once the discharge is complete.

I work to ensure the PCP has the patient summary of care, discharge summary, medication reconciliation list, labs, tests, procedures, follow up plan, and any other relevant information prior to their scheduled appointment. Post discharge, I continually assess and monitor the patient, assist the patient to navigate the healthcare system, appeal health plan denials, make appropriate referrals and address social determinants of health. *See Case Study 4.1: Ensuring Access to Care After Discharge and Case Study 4.2: Best Practices.*

Final Thoughts from the Community Case Manager

Patients are at an increased risk for adverse effects during transitions of care. Best practices for acute case managers to support better patient outcomes when transitioning patients includes assessing patients who are at increased risk, following up on referrals to ensure there are not gaps in care, scheduling outpatient appointments, proving patients resources to make informed choices for quality care, and communicating across the continuum of care.

Case Study 4.1: Ensuring Access to Care After Discharge

Mr. Brown is frequently admitted to the hospital from conditions related to medication non-adherence. His outpatient care team has been working on getting him into an assisted living facility and he previously had medication management through home health. Unfortunately, home health discharged him from service after several months due to his perceived non-adherence. Within two weeks, he was admitted to the hospital due to medication non-adherence. The patient's hospital electronic health record (EHR) listed him as having home health from prior admissions and he was discharged home with a resumption of care order sent to the home health agency. His outpatient care team was unable to reach the patient post discharge.

A couple of weeks later, Mr. Smith was admitted again for the same reason and for the second time, he was discharged back home with a home health resumption of care order placed. By the third admission in six weeks, his outpatient care team did make contact with the case management lead to make her aware the patient was discharged from home health weeks prior so a safe discharge plan could take place.

Communication between inpatient and outpatient teams is imperative for successful transitions of care. If you refer a patient for outpatient services (specialists, DME, home health, etc.), make contact to ensure they can provide care for the patient, accept their insurance, and can meet their needs. The Joint Commission (2016) says "health care organizations can do a better job in contacting the receiving provider to ask what information it needs to receive about a patient to ensure a safe transition." This can be applied to nursing homes, SNFs, home health agencies, assisted living facilities, PCPs, specialists, etc.

It's imperative for CMs to follow the evidence-based strategies discussed previously to improve communication and reduce readmission risk. The value of effective provider communication and use of health technology is immeasurable. It is the case manager's role to prepare the patient for discharge, communicate with the patient, provider, subsequent provider and caregivers (Gillingham, 2020). Patient recovery is usually not complete at discharge and requires ongoing management and follow up after hospital discharge.

Case Study 4.2: Best Practices

Mrs. Smith is a patient with a high utilization pattern. Her PCP visited her at her dialysis facility because she was difficult to contact and had multiple no shows for appointments in the clinic. This patient has not been seen by a PCP at her dialysis facility for several months because the provider's schedule is no longer able to accommodate travel time to the facility. The PCP and her PCP transitions of care (TOC) case manager have been unable to reach her post discharge.

At each admission, health information technology alerts Mrs. Smith's PCP TOC case manager of her admission. The TOC case manager leaves voicemails for Mrs. Smith's hospital case manager at each admission but does not get a call back. Each hospital discharge plan notes the patient's PCP still sees her at the dialysis facility and this is no longer accurate. While the case manager's notes and discharge plan list her PCP by name and location, the patient's EHR is never updated to add PCP information. Summary of cares are never sent to the PCP office because her EHR lists "no PCP on file".

It is critical to assess Mrs. Smith at each admission, update her EHR with the most up to date and accurate information, communicate with her outpatient interdisciplinary care team, and schedule follow up visits prior to patient discharge. These steps are in line with best practices in and would better serve the patient to reduce readmission and decrease high utilization of healthcare resources.

References

Centers for Medicare & Medicaid Services. (2019). CMS; Discharge Planning Rule Supports Interoperability and Patient Preferences. *New protocols improve engagement, choice and continuity of care across hospital settings.*

Code of Federal Regulations, Section 42.483. Centers for Medicare & Medicaid Services, HHS.

Cornett, S. (2009). Assessing and Addressing Health Literacy. *The Online Journal of Issues in Nursing, 14*(3).

Federal Registrar. (2019). Medicare and Medicaid Programs; Revisions to Requirements for Discharge Planning for Hospitals, Critical Access Hospitals, and Home health agencies, and Hospital and Critical Access Hospital Changes to Promote Innovation, Flexibility, and Improvement in Patient Care.

Gillingham, D. C. (2020). CCM Certification Made Easy: Your guide to passing the certified case manager exam. (3rd ed., pp 46). Crestview, FL: Blue Bayou Press, LLC.

Johnson, J. K., Farnan, J. M., Barach, P., Hesselink, G., Wollersheim, Loes Pijnenborg, L., Kalkman, C. & M Arora, V. M. (2012). Searching for the missing pieces between the hospital and primary care: mapping the patient process during care transitions. *BMJ Quality & Safety.*

Kaufman, B. (2016). Readmissions & Medicare: What's the Cost? *NIC Cares Blog.*

Kripalani S., LeFevre F, Phillips C.O., Williams, M. V., Basaviah, P. & Baker, D. B. (2007). Deficits in communication and information transfer between hospital-based and primary care physicians: implications for patient safety and continuity of care. *Journal of the American Medical Association.*

Mansukhani, R. P., Bridgeman, M. B., Candelario, D., Laurie J., & Eckert, L.J. (2015). Exploring Transitional Care: Evidence-Based Strategies for Improving Provider Communication and Reducing Readmissions. *P&T, 40*(10).

Nazir A., Little M.O., & Arling G, W. (2014). More than just location: Helping patients and families select an appropriate skilled nursing facility. *Annals of Long-Term Care: Clinical Care and Aging.*

The Joint Commission. (2016). Transitions of care: The need for collaboration across entire care continuum. *Hot Topics in Health Care*, 2.

The Joint Commission. (2016). Quick Safety 26: Transitions of care: Managing medications.

Tong, L., Arnold, T., Yang, J., Tian, X., Erdmann, C., & Esposito, T. (2018). The association between outpatient follow-up visits and all-cause non-elective 30-day readmissions: A retrospective observational cohort study. *Plos One.*

Tyler, D. A., Gadbois, E. A., McHugh, J. P., Sheild, R. R., Winblad, U. & Mor, V. (2017).

Patients Are Not Given Quality-Of-Care Data About Skilled Nursing Facilities When Discharged From Hospitals. *Health Affairs.*

TRANSITIONS OF CARE: LONG TERM CARE TO COMMUNITY SETTINGS

Tonya Edmonds O'Neil MSN RN CCM

Transitions of care from long term care nursing home facilities back into the community setting can be a challenging experience. Barriers to transition can include unaffordable housing due to a fixed income, caregiver burnout once discharged, and access to community resources. It is imperative to identify those patients who are most suited to transition back to their home, have a natural support system such as family or friends for caregiving, and available resources to sustain their discharge without unnecessary readmissions back to a facility.

When patients are approached by case managers (CMs) regarding their desire to remain in a long-term care nursing facility or transition home, they consistently answer, "I want to go home." Before the CM can start any arrangements for the departure, there are several components to the discharge that must be handled. There needs to be an organized plan for the transition to home and the decision to return home should not be made lightly. Rushing to discharge a patient for any reason can cause an unsafe discharge, unnecessary readmission, or could even be fatal.

Properly transitioning patients from long term care back to the community is a collaborative process where all parties are equally indebted to the success of the discharge. The goal is to discharge a patient physically and medically ready to return to the comforts of their own home with family or friends. Effective and safe transitions to home allows nursing homes the space to utilize a bed for another patient who needs that level of care.

Background

According to a Harris-Kogetin (2016), a National Study on long term care providers between the years of 2013 to 2014, there were roughly 65,600 regulated long-term care providers paid to provide adult day care centers, home health agencies, hospices, assisted living facilities, residential care facilities, and nursing homes. Of those paid providers 15,600 of them were nursing homes that had a capacity of 1,660,400 licensed maximum beds. Out of 1,347,600 long term care residents of nursing facilities, 16.5% were under the age of 65 and 83.5% were over 65 years old. In addition to requiring assistance with activities daily of living (ADLs), they also were diagnosed with several different chronic or debilitating diseases such as Alzheimer's Disease, chronic obstructive pulmonary disease, arthritis, asthma, chronic kidney disease, depression, diabetes, hypertension, and osteoporosis.

These nursing home residents had an average length of stay (LOS) of about 485 days and of those days, 57% of them were long-term care residents (Harris-Kogetin et al., 2016). "The current growth of the population ages 65 and older is one of the most significant demographic trends in the history of the United States" (Mather, Jacobsen, & Pollard, 2015). With the increase in our older population there comes a life expectancy of older adults living to be a lot older. According to the U.S. Census Bureau there has been a steady increase in the number of Americans living longer. It is estimated the current population of 46 million seniors over the age of 65, will more than double from 2014 to 2060 (Mather, Jacobsen, & Pollard, 2015).

Barriers

The increase in the number of older Americans can also increase the number of residents in long term care facilities who will require assistance in transitioning back into the community. It is crucial for CMs to understand these trends and be prepared to anticipate the needs of their patients. Residents of these facilities have a variety of illnesses that require assistance upon discharge. Most of them will return home with minimal to significant personal care assistance with their ADLs. It is imperative for CMs to carefully assess the amount of assistance that will dictate the appropriate level of care for discharge to home. If the need for assistance at home is too great, transitioning out of the facility may not be a viable option. Therefore, the decision needs to be a collaborative effort with members of the transition of care team.

There are patients currently residing in long term care that have completely recovered from the acute illness that landed them there in the first place. They are highly functional independent patients who require very little if any personal care assistance upon discharge. Their major barrier is insufficient availability to affordable housing. If there are no family members prepared to offer a place to stay, these residents are forced to stay at a facility where they are not at the appropriate level of care. The CM and social services department need to work in tandem with local county professionals to determine when affordable housing becomes available. The Managed Care Organization (MCO) assigned field or telephonic care coordinators can assist in locating affordable housing for these members as well.

According to the U. S. Department of Housing and Urban Development Public Housing Voucher Program (2021) there are opportunities for income-based housing that provide affordable rent prices for individuals who need them. Unfortunately, because of the high demand for these apartments, there are also very long waitlists that are not always open. The CM can work with the social worker or MCO care coordinator in getting patients added to these wait lists as they become open and monitor for when an apartment is available.

The patients who are interested in discharging from nursing facilities back home may require a great deal of assistance with their ADLs upon discharge. The patient could have chronic illnesses that need to be monitored, debilitating diseases that will only progress over time, or functional limitations that are irreversible. These patients are usually discharged back to the home they left, home with family, or to senior apartments.

Patients who transitioned from the Medicare SNF to the Medicaid long-term care bed can also qualify for home care. This transition supports caregivers that are utilizing MCO Medicaid Waiver caregiver services. This is dependent on the patient's income and CMs should also determine if there are any out-of-pocket expenses. These services can be agency directed care where the caregiver is provided by the agency. Consumer directed care is when the caregiver is a family or friend who gets paid to provide the personal care assistance. Prior to discharge the CM will assess the patient needs, determine where they will be discharged to, and identify who will provide that service (Department of Medical Assistance Medicaid for Virginia, 2021).

The Team

Beginning the process of a successful transition back home starts with communication. The CM must communicate with the patient to identify if they are interested in discharging. The nursing facility's minimum data set (MDS) form is a great way to identify which patients are interested in discharging because it assesses the patient's functional status and desire to go home. Once it is determined that a patient wants to begin the process of being discharged, the family should be brought into the conversation. It is important that someone from the family who lives near the patient is identified as this patient's natural support in case of an emergency, to provide care when the agency caregiver is not available, and to assist in coordination care for the patient's discharge. However, there are times when the patients are cognitively intact whom request to discharge without a natural support. The nursing facility is required to adhere to the patient's request. The transition care team may include the nursing facility social worker, MCO care coordinator, family, community department of health case worker, and the patient.

The Paperwork

Please note the process may differ slightly from state to state. This example illustrates the process in Virginia. Whether the patient is discharging home with or without waiver services there are forms that need to be completed per the Department of Medical Assistance Services (DMAS). If a patient does not require personal care assistance and are considered community well, they only need to have the DMAS 80 Nursing Facility Admission, Discharge, or Level of Care Change form. If they need personal care assistance, several other forms are required:

- DMAS 99 Community-Based Care Individual Assessment Report
- DMAS 98 R Home and Community Based Services Request Form
- DMAS 97 A/B Provider Plan of Care
- DMAS 80 Nursing Facility Admission, Discharge or Level of Care Change

Upon admission to the nursing facility a document called a Uniform Assessment Inventory (UAI) is completed. Usually, this assessment takes place at the hospital to determine the need for a SNF level of care. It is used at discharge to determine if the patient qualifies for Home and Community Based Services (HCBS). The UAI can also be performed at the nursing home. If that is not possible, the local health department and DHS can perform this assessment. "HCBS waivers are designed to meet the needs of people who prefer to get long-term care services and supports in their home or community, rather than in an institutional setting" (Department of Medical Assistance Services Medicaid for Virginia, 2021). These documents are examined and used to help determine how many hours are needed for caregiver services.

The Transition to Community

If the patient qualifies for the Medicaid waiver program, the team continues to move forward with the discharge. A primary care provider (PCP) is identified, DME that was ordered is scheduled for delivery, transportation is arranged, and the home is prepared for the arrival. The planning for a patient to return home does not just stop at the facility. Planning also includes the community in which the patient must live.

The MCO care coordinator must assess the home to determine that it is a safe environment for the patient to return. The community is also assessed for additional resources such as delivered meals, pharmacy delivery, ongoing transportation, and the essential utilities are set up. The transition team needs to determine if home health services are needed such as nursing or therapy services. If so, those orders need to be sent over to the desired home health agency intact coordinator to prompt a care visit to be arranged soon after the patient gets discharged. Appointments need to be set up with PCPs to happen with 30 days of discharge if not sooner.

Once at home, the patient needs to be followed closely by contacting them several times during the first week, then weekly, monthly, and as needed. There are a lot of challenges during the first 30 days of discharge. If the patient qualifies for Medicaid waiver services, they will be assigned a care coordinator by the MCO who will ensure all needs are met for the duration of their care at home. Checking in with the patient ensures that all scheduled services are happening, periodic health risk assessments are done, and any outstanding issues are resolved.

Caregivers are assessed for caregiver burnout. The causes of caregiver burnout may include but not limited to the emotional impact of the patient's condition, conflicting demands trying to juggle other responsibilities, increased workload, and lack of privacy (Fisher, 2020). The community-based CM needs to be keenly aware of these symptoms that may require further discussion with the caregiver such as depression, withdrawal, feelings of helplessness, negative emotions, physical fatigue, abuse, neglect, personal health problems, and low self-esteem. There are online resources and community resources available that can support individuals with caregiver burnout symptoms. An in-depth assessment of all community resources applicable to this patient's individualized needs should be identified with appropriate referrals.

Impact of COVID-19 on Transitions of Care

There are avoidable obstacles that can be managed when transitioning patients from a nursing facility to home. During the COVID-19 pandemic, transitions of care services have been even more complicated. There can be numerous factors that negatively impact patients who desire to transition home. According to a health and science news report on CNBC (2020), nursing homes have become ground zero for COVID-19 outbreaks across the United States where the most vulnerable members of our society live.

A COVID-19 Tracking Project stated "there have been more than 33.9 million confirmed U.S. coronavirus cases with at least 607,000 deaths as of July 12, 2021. Of those who died, 30.3% or 167,000 cases have been in long term care facilities (AARP, 2021). Family members were becoming desperate to get their loved ones out of nursing homes as soon as possible. When patients were discharged without proper planning, the transition team was not prepared to assist in a safe discharge. Often the MCO care coordinators were notified after the discharge happened because the nursing facilities were so overwhelmed with patient care. When unplanned discharges happen, patients can be at risk for readmission to acute care facilities for falls, improper medication reconciliation, exacerbation of chronic illnesses, or even worse outcomes.

Conclusion

Transitioning home from a nursing facility is a collaborative effort that starts with the patient. If managed properly, the patient will return home to a safe, supportive, and loving environment. The members of the transition team can vary depending on the availability of staff and resources. When transitioned correctly, the collaborative effort is more likely to be successful, and the return home can happen without any untoward negative setbacks. Building a strong transition care team that extend past the walls of the facility out into the community is the only way to provide the post discharge care needed to secure a sustainable return home.

References

AARP. (2021). AARP Nursing Home COVID-19 Dashboard.

Department of Medical Assistance Services Medicaid for Virginia. (n.d.).

Fisher, M. (2020, June 25). Causes and Symptoms of Caregiver Burnout: Called to Care: Johns Hopkins Bayview Medical Center in Baltimore, MD.

Harris-Kogetin, L., Park-Lee, E., Sengupta, M., Caffrey, C., Rome, V., & Lendon, J. (2016). Long-Term Care Providers and Services Users in the United States: Data From the National Study of Long-Term Care Providers, 2013–2014. *National Center for Health Statistics, 43*(3).

Housing Choice Vouchers Fact Sheet. (n.d.).

Mather, M., Jacobsen, L., & Pollard, K. (2015). Aging in the United States. *Population Reference Bureau*, 70(2).

Stankiewicz, K. & Rattner, N. (2020, December 02). Nursing homes create 'perfect storm' for COVID outbreaks as cases and deaths surge again.

COLLABORATIONS WITH MANAGED CARE CASE MANAGERS

Deanna Cooper Gillingham RN CCM

Have you ever wished you had your own personal contact at the insurance company? Someone to help you navigate the system, and to work with you to get your patient the services they need? Someone to collaborate with on discharge planning (which we all know begins on admission)? Someone who understands how the insurance company works, the needs of the patient, and can guide you through the maze of departments and paperwork? Well for your most complex patients you do have a resource, and that person is the managed care case manager.

Think of the managed care case manager (CM) as an extension of your staff that works at the managed care company, for the specific client they are assigned to. This person can be called on to help with discharge planning, medication issues, DME acquisition, extracontractual benefits, transportation issues, caregiver support, appeals for denied services, and patient/caregiver education among other things.

The CM can answer questions such as:

- Does this patient qualify for SNF or rehab?
- How can we expedite discharge planning?
- Which home health company did they use previously?
- Which medications are formulary?
- How can approval for a specialty pharmacy item be obtained?
- Are there resources for non-formulary medications?
- Does DME, outpatient procedure, surgery, etc. require prior authorization?
- What information needs to be submitted to obtain authorization?
- What information is needed to submit an appeal and have the best chance of approval?
- And so much more!

CMs can begin to assist you as soon as the patient is admitted (or before for scheduled procedures and admissions) and their help can continue long after the patient is discharged (decreasing those 30-day readmission rates). By contacting the CM when the patient is admitted you can collaborate on a discharge plan. The CM can follow the patient through the hospital stay with your assistance, collecting the clinical information needed to approve the discharge plan. Then, when the patient is ready to discharge, the approval can come as quickly as a phone call!

By sharing discharge instructions with the CM, you provide them with the information they need to support the patient after discharge. Is the patient discharging home with home care? The CM can follow up to make sure the patient is admitted to home care without a hitch. Was DME ordered?

The CM can make sure there are no issues with its arrival or use. Is the patient unable to drive? Do they have follow-up appointments and prescriptions to fill? The CM can follow up after discharge to make sure the medications have been received and are being taken properly. They can also call the patient a day or two before the follow-up appointment to make sure they have transportation.

CMs also check medication compliance by making sure the medications are filled on a routine basis. They routinely reconcile medications from all providers reporting any discrepancies as well as checking for any barriers to taking the medication as prescribed such as side effects, trouble filling the medication, or remembering to take the medication. CMs also provide and/or reinforce medication teaching. All of this helps decrease readmissions. *See Case Study 4.3.*

We all know it is not quite as simple as this scenario played out. There is a lot of work done behind the scenes by everyone involved. The point is that when everyone works together, everyone's job is easier and the patient's results are greatly improved.

I do not want to give the impression that CMs are miracle workers. Each medical policy is different, with different benefits and restrictions. The CM is the person who best knows the available benefits and resources of each policy. I encourage you to respond to contacts from the CM and ask how they can help you to help the client.

Tips for working with CMs:

- If you have a patient that you feel would benefit from case management, reach out to the managed care company to see if this member can have a CM
- Involve the CM as early as possible
- Share information including clinical, potential problems, complications, support systems, social determinants of health (SDoH), and other information that will help them to understand the situation better. You are their eyes and ears.
- Remember you are both on the same team, "Team Patient"
- Call them back because they are trying to help your patient
- Encourage patient to work with case management
- Make part of your initial assessment the question "are you working with or have you worked with a case manager at the insurance company?"

Case Study 4.3

Mr. Brody is a 54-year-old diabetic who is a frequent visitor to your emergency department (ED). He has been admitted for uncontrolled blood sugars three times in the last seven months. He misses his doctor appointments. His blood sugars are not under control and he has now developed a non-healing foot ulcer. He complains that he does not have reliable transportation to his medical appointments and does not routinely check his blood sugar because "those strips cost too much."

You receive a voicemail from the insurance company CM, Mary, who has been assigned to his case. She requests a callback to discuss Mr. Brody's needs. When you call her back, she explains that she has been assigned Mr. Brody's case due to the request for a wound vac and multiple ED visits. She has been unable to reach him by phone. You explain to her that Mr. Brody is nonadherent to his medical regimen and explain his reasons why.

Mary informs you that Mr. Brody is eligible for the diabetic coaching program, which includes free blood sugar testing supplies, waived copays on diabetic medications, as well as education. There is also a transportation assistance program available to him which will provide transportation to and from medical appointments. She would be happy to enroll him in these programs but will need to speak to him. You agree to connect Mr. Brody with the CM and to encourage him to return her calls so that he can enroll in the case management program to receive these benefits.

Next, Mary discusses with you the required documentation she needs to approve the wound vac. She requests that you fax it directly to her so that she can handle it personally and expedite the approval.

In this scenario, everyone wins. Mr. Brody now has the resources he needs to manage his diabetes, adhere to the plan of care, and heal his diabetic foot ulcer. You are able to get approval for the needed resources quickly and decrease future ED visits and admissions. The managed care company is happy that his blood sugars are under control and his wound is healing, saving them the cost of future complications from diabetes.

CONNECTION WITH MANAGED CARE CASE MANAGERS

Cassandra Battle BSN RN

Each practice setting has its own unique structure, features, and financial incentives that shape the practice of medicine and case management. The goal of health insurance case management is to make patient transitions as efficiently and economically as possible. The case manager (CM) also anticipates the patient's future health care needs and tries to put in place mechanisms to meet those needs as efficiently as possible. The health insurance company's CM receives information from hospital CMs, home health care companies, physician's offices, social workers, and other health care providers. Depending on the insurer and the location, the CM may even visit a patient in the hospital. Because CMs work for health insurance companies, hospitals, and other providers, they attempt to keep costs down as much as possible. With rising costs in healthcare, case management can be a useful tool for both consumers and companies alike.

The Process

The best way to collaborate with other professional disciplines is to know the role of the other professional. One of the largest case management settings is Managed Care Case Management. These CMs work within insurance agencies. There are multiple sub settings within managed care. Examples include disease management, critical care CMs, quality assurance case management, and utilization case management. All play a part in patient-centric goals.

Let's look at how it works. The patient is enrolled onto a disease management case load. This process consists of a disease manager (DM) who conducts a health risk assessment by motivational interviewing. DMs determine if the patient has any needs that can be managed by a DM such as:

- Depression
- Bipolar
- Schizophrenia
- Substance use
- Alzheimer's, dementia
- Asthma, COPD
- CAD, CHF, hypertension (HTN)
- Diabetes
- HIV/AIDS
- Obesity or overweight
- Adolescent depression

The DM creates a plan of care with the patient. If the patient has an acute flare up and must be admitted into an acute care setting, the DM case manager collaborates with the acute CM to assure safe and efficient care along the continuum. *See Case Study 4.4.*

Case Study 4.4

Ms. Harris is a 56-year female who was initially enrolled onto a DM caseload three months ago. The DM stratifies the patient as a level two. This level includes a monthly DM contact to the patient to review and assess goals. Ms. Harris usually reports that her overall condition is good, but sometimes fair. Her Patient Health Questionnaire-2 (PHQ2) depression screening was self-reported as two. (Note: The PHQ-2 is a two question first step screening. Patients who screen positive (score of three (3) or more), should be evaluated using the more detailed Patient Health Questionnaire-9 (PHQ-9) (American Psychological Association, 2011). She presents with diabetes and her most recent HgbA1c is 11.2%. She also reports a history of HTN, CHF, and COPD. She also reports that she smokes half of a pack of cigarettes a day. Ms. Harris reports to the DM that she was just in the emergency room because she was having a hard time breathing.

During this monthly call, Ms. Harris voiced that she was glad the DM called because she was thinking about going back to the emergency room. The DM asked the patient what her concerns were and why she felt that she needed to go the emergency room. Ms. Harris voiced that she has not seen her doctor since her last hospital visit due to the COVID-19 pandemic. She explained that she was extremely fearful about going into the doctor's office or the hospital. Ms. Harris also shared with the DM that she had increased the number of daily cigarettes she smoked to a pack and a half.

Ms. Harris told the DM that she has not been 'doing her daily blood sugars' and has been having a hard time controlling her diet because 'all she does is sit at home and eat because she cannot go out because of covid. The DM noted audible wheezing during the conversation. The DM asked if Ms. Harris would mind checking her blood sugar while on the phone because Ms. Harris could not remember her last blood sugar. Ms. Harris agreed and her blood sugar monitor read HI. Ms. Harris reported swelling in her hands, feet, and ankles. The DM asked Ms. Harris if she were willing to see her primary care doctor if she could secure an appointment. She agreed and the DM completed a conference call with the patient's primary care office, but the office had special hours due to the COVID-19 pandemic.

Ms. Harris was in agreement that she needed to go to the emergency room (ER) since coordination with her primary care office could not be achieved. The patient's son was available to take her to the ER. The DM assured Ms. Harris that she would call ahead of time to speak with ER staff members to let them know that Ms. Harris was on the way by private vehicle. The DM provided a brief report and requested the acute care CM contact her once the patient was assigned. The DM did receive a call back from the acute CM.

During this introduction call, the DM was reassured the acute CM had the patient's current and correct medication list, history of diagnosis, and brief medical history of patient based on previous interaction with the DM. The DM informed the acute CM the patient lived alone, however, her son is nearby for emergencies. Ms. Harris's blood pressure on arrival was 198/102, blood sugar was 543 and she was in acute congestive heart failure (CHF) with exacerbation of chronic obstructive pulmonary disease (COPD). The plan was to stabilize the patient and discharge her home with connection to her primary care office.

However, discharging her home would mean that she would need to weigh herself daily, check her daily blood sugars, self-administer her medications as prescribed, and demonstrate proper use of her inhaler. Identified gaps in care included further education for the need of tobacco cessation and healthier eating, diet, and lifestyle changes. The DM collaborated with the acute CM to set the patient up with follow up primary care visits, a dietician, other support services, and ensure that she had working glucometer machine and weight scale at home. Ms. Harris was discharged on home after a three day stay in the hospital.

The acute CM contacted the DM to inform of the patient's discharge and discharge plan. The DM contacted the patient the same day and based on the recent hospitalization and information received, re-stratified the patient as level three—which included more frequent patient contact to every two weeks. Currently, Ms. Harris has improved in her self-management skills. She has been able to make and attend her scheduled primary care visits. Her medications have been adjusted. She keeps a log of daily blood sugars, weights, and blood pressures. Tobacco cessation and nutrition classes and support groups have been initiated. This collaboration of Disease Manager CM and the acute CM was successful.

Chapter 5:

Compliance and Medicare Rules and Notices

UNDERSTANDING YOUR PATIENT'S INSURANCE BENEFITS

It is important to have a thorough knowledge of the patient's insurance coverage, what benefits available, and any limitations of their particular plan's coverage. This is markedly important when coordinating care across the continuum.

- Does the plan cover the recommended level of post-acute care?
    - There are plans that do not cover certain levels of care, such as Inpatient Rehabilitation Facility (IRF) or Skilled Nursing Facility/Sub-Acute Rehabilitation (SNF/SAR).
    - Some plans must negotiate all post-acute transitions on an individual case-by-case basis. Know the plans you work with most frequently to gain a working understanding of the transitional care benefits available.
    - When in doubt, make sure to connect with the plan CM to collaborate on transition planning.
- What are the in-network versus out-of-network resources available and potentials costs to the patient?
    - Again, your best resource is the plan CM.
    - Familiarize yourself with the various plans' websites. You can find benefit information, formularies, and utilize search engines for in-network resources (physicians, post-acute care providers, pharmacies, etc.)
- Does the plan's formulary cover the medications prescribed?
    - Plan formularies are available on their websites.

MEDICARE BENEFITS (DAYS, CO-INSURANCE, AND LIFETIME RESERVE DAYS)

When working with Medicare beneficiaries, there are important details to remember regarding benefits available. An excellent resource to review all Medicare benefits and the criteria to access is Medicare Interactive at https://www.medicareinteractive.org/get-answers/medicare-covered-services.

Medicare Part A (hospital insurance) covers inpatient hospital care when the patient is admitted to the hospital as an inpatient and the hospital accepts Medicare. Inpatient hospital care includes care can be used in the following facility types:

- Acute care hospitals
- Critical access hospitals
- Inpatient rehabilitation facilities

- Inpatient psychiatric facilities
- Long-term care hospitals
- Inpatient care as part of a qualifying clinical research study

Benefit periods are used to measure the patient's use of inpatient hospital and skilled nursing facility (SNF) services. By Medicare's definition, a benefit period begins the day the patient is admitted to a hospital as an inpatient, or to a SNF, and ends the day when the patient has been out of the hospital or SNF for 60 days in a row. This is also referred to as an "episode of care" (Centers for Medicare and Medicaid, 2019).

Costs borne by the patient under Medicare include:

- Hospital Days 1–60: $0 coinsurance for each benefit period.
- Hospital Days 61–90: $352 coinsurance per day of each benefit period.
- Hospital Days 91 and beyond: $704 coinsurance per each "lifetime reserve day" after day 90 for each benefit period (up to 60 days over the patient's lifetime).
- Beyond lifetime reserve days: all costs.
- Inpatient mental health care in a psychiatric hospital is limited to 190 days in a lifetime.
- (Centers for Medicare and Medicaid, 2019).

If the patient has used their 90 days of hospital coverage but needs to stay longer, Medicare covers up to 60 additional benefit days, called "lifetime reserve days", for which they will pay a daily coinsurance. These days are nonrenewable, meaning the patient will not get them back when they become eligible for another benefit period (Medicare Interactive, 2021).

Medicare will stop paying for inpatient-related hospital costs (such as room and board) if the patient "runs out of days" during the benefit period. To be eligible for a new benefit period and additional days of inpatient coverage, the patient must remain out of the hospital or SNF for 60 days in a row (Medicare Interactive, 2021).

References

Centers for Medicare and Medicaid. (2019). Hospital Inpatient Care Coverage.

Medicare Interactive. (2021). Medicare Part A Covered Services.

Resources

Medicare Interactive at https://www.medicareinteractive.org/get-answers/medicare-covered-services

MEDICARE COMPLIANCE FORMS

In regards to Medicare, compliance addresses notification of the Medicare beneficiary the patient's rights, and transparency of potential beneficiary financial responsibility. Medicare has developed several forms to be utilized in an effort to standardize the information presented and the overall notification process.

Medicare Forms include:

- **MOON/NOON**: Medicare Outpatient Observation Notice/Non-Medicare Outpatient Observation Notice (by state, if required)
- **IMM**: Important Message from Medicare
- **HINN**: Hospital Issued Notice of Noncoverage
- **ABN**: Advanced Beneficiary Notice
- **Patient Choice**: not a Medicare issued form, however, this is a Medicare Compliance issue

General Information About Medicare Form Completion

Any Medicare Notice must be:

1. Given by a person or entity designated by Medicare as a "notifier." These designated notifiers include physicians, providers (including facilities and their representatives), practitioners, hospice providers, home health agencies, and suppliers.
2. Reviewed verbally with the beneficiary or representative, giving an opportunity for questions to be answered prior to signing.
3. Delivered far enough in advance that the beneficiary or representative has time to consider the options and make an informed choice.
4. Signed by the beneficiary or representative and a copy provided.
5. A copy of the signed completed form retained in the patient's file.

Signature/Attestation/Alternative Delivery Models

Applicable to all Medicare notices, in cases where the beneficiary may not be able to receive, comprehend, or sign the notice being presented, there are alternative means of delivery allowed by CMS. The process follows and is applicable to all Medicare notices listed above.

If the beneficiary is unable to comprehend the notice, the notice must be delivered to the beneficiary's representative to be signed within two business days. A representative is an individual who, under state or other applicable law, may make healthcare decisions on a beneficiary's behalf (e.g., the beneficiary's legal guardian, or someone appointed in accordance with a properly executed "durable medical power of attorney"). This person (typically, a family member or close friend) is someone whom the beneficiary has indicated may make decisions, but who has not been named in any legal or binding document. This type of individual may be a representative for purpose of receiving this notice. Such representatives must have the patient's best interest at heart and must act in a manner that is protective of the beneficiary's rights.

If the beneficiary is incapable of or incompetent to receive the notice, and the hospital cannot obtain the signature of the beneficiary's representative, a hospital representative should telephone the beneficiary's representative to advise the beneficiary's rights as a hospital patient, including the right to appeal a discharge decision.

1. The date of receipt of the notices is the date when the hospital conveys this information to the representative, whether in writing or by telephone.

2. The mailing address of the beneficiary's representative should be obtained. Document confirmation of speaking with the representative by mailing the original copy of the form to the beneficiary's representative on the same date.

3. Place a dated copy of the notice in the beneficiary's medical record and document the telephone conversation with the beneficiary's representative on the notice.

4. The documentation should also include the name of the staff person initiating the contact, the name of the representative contacted by phone, the date and the time of the telephone contact, and the telephone number called.

When direct phone contact cannot be made, the hospital representative should send the original copy of the notice to the beneficiary's representative by certified mail and return receipt requested It is important to include documentation on the notice of attempted phone calls including dates and times of the calls, the name of the staff person who attempted the calls, and the name and phone number of the representative they attempted to reach.

Documentation the notice was sent should include the name of the staff person who sent the notice, the name and address of the representative to whom the notice was sent and the date and time it was sent. The date received is the date that someone at the representative's address signs (or refuses to sign) the receipt. Remember to place a copy in the return receipt in the beneficiary's medical record.

MEDICARE OUTPATIENT OBSERVATION NOTICE (MOON)

Observation services have been around for a long time. The problem is that patients and their families haven't always been notified when they were in observation status. From their perspectives, there may be no noticeable difference between time in the hospital as an inpatient or in observation status. Medicare considers observation care to be an outpatient service. Subsequently, patients who are classified as outpatients in the hospital may face unforeseen complications of a potential discharge plan or financial consequences post-hospitalization. They may fail to meet the three-day inpatient stay guidelines to qualify for Medicare coverage for SNF stay. Patients in observation status may also have higher co-payments and charges for doctors' fees, hospital services, and medications.

In response to these issues and advocacy by several groups on behalf of the Medicare population, CMS released the Medicare Outpatient Observation Notice (MOON) form. The intent of the form is to educate Medicare beneficiaries on their status as an outpatient versus inpatient, the related impact to their out-of-pocket expenses as an outpatient, and the potential impact of their observation status on out-of-pocket expenses if they are released to a SNF.

Timeframes for Delivery

All acute care facilities must provide the MOON form to Medicare beneficiaries receiving outpatient observation services for more than 24 hours and within 36 hours of the patient receiving outpatient observation services (or sooner if released). The form must be signed by the beneficiary or representative. There must be an oral explanation to the beneficiary along with the form. Failure to provide the MOON is a violation of the hospital's Medicare provider agreement, which could result in the termination of that agreement.

Completion of the MOON Form

Completion of the MOON form should follow the standard guidelines outlines in the "General Information About Medicare Form Completion" at the beginning of this chapter. There are two sections that require explanations to be inserted. The explanations are to be delivered verbally to the patient or their representative. If the patient is not able to receive or defers to their representative, then the form must be signed by the representative or there must be documentation present stating if a patient or representative declines to sign.

"You're a hospital outpatient receiving observation services. You are not an inpatient because:"

Fill in the specific reason the patient is in an outpatient status, rather than an inpatient stay. Use easy to read, plain language to explain why the patient is in observation status versus inpatient.

"Additional Information:"

Any additional information that would be helpful to the patient can be included here. Examples include: Accountable Care Organization (ACO) information, notation that a beneficiary refused to sign the notice, any waivers or cost sharing responsibilities that may impact the patient's financial responsibility, or contact information for physicians, financial office, or others that would be useful to the patient.

References

Centers for Medicare & Medicaid. (2018). Medicare Outpatient Observation Notice.

Hirsch, R. (2016). 10 things to know about MOON: The Medicare Outpatient Observation Notice.

Kipple, J. (2017). CMS Medicare Outpatient Observation Notice (MOON) Form.

Takacs McGinnis Elder Care Law. (2018). What You Need to Know about the MOON.

Resources

Medicare MOON Form https://www.cms.gov/Medicare/Medicare-General-Information/BNI/MOON

IMPORTANT MESSAGE FROM MEDICARE (IMM)

Background

Medicare beneficiaries who are hospital inpatients have a statutory right to appeal to a Medicare Quality Improvement Organization (QIO) for an expedited review when a hospital, with physician concurrence, determines that inpatient care is no longer necessary. These regulations are referenced at 42 CFR 489.27 and 412.42 (c)(3). The authority for these instructions stems from Sections 1866(a)(1)(M), 1869(c)(3)(C)(iii)(III), and 1154(e) of the Social Security Act (Centers for Medicare and Medicaid, 2018).

All Medicare inpatients will receive the Important Message from Medicare (IMM) at admission and discharge as required by CMS regulations. The IMM notifies the patient of their hospital discharge appeal rights. Delivery of this form and the accompanying documentation ensures that all hospital inpatients are notified about their discharge appeal rights.

The IMM is given only to Medicare beneficiaries who have an inpatient admission order. Observation patients are not inpatients and are considered outpatients. They do not have the appeal rights outlined in the IMM.

Education and Delivery

Initial Notice

Hospital representatives must provide the IMM at or near admission, but no later than two calendar days from the day of admission. Another option is to deliver it at preadmission, but not more than seven calendar days before admission. A patient's or representative's signature and date must be obtained to indicate receipt of notice. The original is given to the patient with a copy retained by the hospital for the patient's electronic health records.

The responsibility for delivery of the IMM does not stop at delivery and obtaining of signatures. The hospital representative is responsible for explaining the beneficiary's rights of discharge appeal under Medicare and should be able to answer any questions the patient or family may have pertaining to those rights.

Follow-Up Notice

The follow-up IMM is required for lengths of stay greater than two days and must also be provided to the patient as soon as possible prior to discharge, but no more than two days before. When a discharge seems likely within one to two days, the follow-up notice should be given to the patient in an appropriate amount of time to allow the patient ample time to review and act on it.

When the discharge cannot be predicted in advance, the follow-up copy of the notice may be delivered as late as the day of discharge. If the follow-up copy of the notice must be delivered on the day of discharge, hospitals must give beneficiaries who need it at least four hours to consider their right to request a QIO review. Beneficiaries may choose to leave prior to that time; however, hospitals must not pressure a beneficiary to leave during this period.

Caveats

- If the hospital delivers the follow-up notice, and the beneficiary status subsequently changes so the discharge is beyond the two-day timeframe, hospitals must deliver another copy of the signed notice again within two calendar days of the new planned discharge date.

- A follow-up copy is not required prior to transfers from one inpatient hospital setting to another inpatient hospital setting (for example, a short-term acute care hospital to a long-term acute care hospital).

- A follow-up copy of the signed notice is required prior to discharge to a lower level of care, such as a SNF.

If the beneficiary refuses to sign the IMM, hospitals may annotate the notice to indicate the refusal, and the date of refusal is considered the date of receipt of the notice. The annotation may be placed in the unused patient signature line, in the "Additional Information" section on page two of the notice or another sheet of paper may be attached to the notice. The hospital must give the original copy of the signed or annotated notice to the patient.

Discharge Appeal Process

If a beneficiary disagrees with the discharge, they can request an expedited appeal (the right to appeal a discharge decision) and contact their QIO.

1. The QIO will contact the hospital to request medical records. After the QIO has contacted the hospital, the CM should complete the Detailed Notice of Discharge, make a copy, and provide the patient with the original copy of the Detailed Notice of Discharge. The CM should provide the QIO with the information they have requested.

2. Patients may not be involuntarily discharged or billed for additional days while an appeal is pending.

3. If the QIO upholds the appropriateness of the discharge, the beneficiary's liability for continued services begins at noon of the day after the QIO notifies the beneficiary and after they are given a Hospital Issued Notice of Non-coverage (HINN).

4. If the QIO upholds the decision to terminate services or discharge the beneficiary, the beneficiary may request expedited reconsideration, orally or in writing, by noon of the calendar day following the QIO's initial notification. The reconsideration will be conducted by the QIC, which must issue a decision within 72 hours of the request. If the QIC does not comply with the time frame, the beneficiary may "escalate" the case to the administrative law judge level.

Best Practices

CMS does not recommend delivering the IMM multiple times during the patient's stay to ensure compliance with the delivery timeline outlined above. Use your clinical judgment to forecast when your patient may be approaching discharge to ensure the delivery within the mandated guidelines. Hospitals may not develop procedures for delivery of the follow-up copy routinely on the day of discharge.

References

Centers for Medicare and Medicaid. (2018). CoP §482.13(a)(1) https://www.cms.gov/Regulations-and-Guidance/Guidance/Transmittals/downloads/R37SOMA.pdf

Centers for Medicare and Medicaid. (2018). Medicare Claims Processing Manual, Chapter 30, Financial Liability Protections at Section 200 and Important Message from Medicare.

Moore, F. (2018). NAHAM Launches Its Key Issues Monitoring Program: Taking a Closer Look at the IM and the MOON. https://www.naham.org/page/Connections-Taking-a-Look-at-the-IM-and-MOON

Resources

Medicare Important Message from Medicare Forms and Instructions https://www.cms.gov/regulations-and-guidance/guidance/transmittals/downloads/r1257cp.pdf

ADVANCE BENEFICIARY NOTICE OF NONCOVERAGE (ABN)

Overview

The Advance Beneficiary Notice of Non-coverage (ABN) is a notice given to beneficiaries (patients) to convey that Medicare is not likely to provide coverage in a specific case. An ABN is a Medicare waiver of liability that providers are required to give a Medicare patient for services provided that may not be covered or considered medically necessary.

This notice must be delivered prior to providing the services because it transfers the potential financial liability to the beneficiary or patient. The Medicare notification process outlined earlier is followed for delivery.

The ABN may also be used to provide notification of financial liability for items or services that Medicare never covers. When the ABN is used in this way, it is not necessary for the beneficiary to choose an option box or sign the notice.

Completing the Notice

ABNs must be printed on a single page. The notifier information (name, address, phone, ID number) and the beneficiary or patient information (name, patient identifier) must be included. Do not use the patient's Medicare number or social security number on this form.

The notifier must list the specific names of the items or services believed to be non-covered. If there is a partial denial, be specific about the exact component of the service expected to be denied. For services that may be repeated or considered a continuous care, denote the frequency or duration of the service. General descriptions are allowed and itemized lists are not required.

The rationale for "why Medicare may not pay" must be documented in easy to understand, lay terms. There must be at least one reason applicable to each item or service listed. Examples of reasons for non-coverage include:

- "Medicare does not pay for this test for your condition."
- "Medicare does not pay for this test as often as this (denied as too frequent)."
- "Medicare does not pay for experimental or research use tests."

The beneficiary or patient must be provided with a reasonable estimate for all of the items or services that are listed as the beneficiary's potential financial responsibility. Multiple items or services that are routinely grouped can be bundled into a single cost estimate.

Patient Decision

- Option 1: This option allows the beneficiary to receive the items and/or services at issue and requires the notifier to submit a claim to Medicare. This will result in a payment decision that can be appealed.

- Option 2: This option allows the beneficiary to receive the non-covered items and/or services and pay for them out of pocket. No claim will be filed and Medicare will not be billed. Therefore, there are no appeal rights associated with this option.

- Option 3: This option means the beneficiary does not want the care in question. By checking this box, the beneficiary understands that no additional care will be provided, and there are no appeal rights associated with this option.

The beneficiary or their representative must choose only one of the three options listed. If there are multiple items or services listed and the beneficiary wants to receive some, but not all of the items or services, the notifier can accommodate this request by using more than one ABN. The notifier can furnish an additional ABN listing the items or services the beneficiary wishes to receive with the corresponding option. If the beneficiary cannot or will not make a choice, the notice should be annotated ("beneficiary refused to choose an option").

The Additional Information section can be used by notifiers to provide additional clarification such as:

- A statement advising the beneficiary to notify his or her provider about certain tests that were ordered, but not received

- Information on other insurance coverage for beneficiaries, such as a Medigap policy (if applicable)

- An additional dated witness signature

- Other necessary annotations

References

Centers for Medicare and Medicaid. (2018). Fee For Service Advanced Beneficiary Notice.

Resources

Medicare Advanced Beneficiary Notice Form and Instructions https://www.cms.gov/Medicare/Medicare-General-Information/BNI/ABN

HOSPITAL ISSUED NOTICE OF NONCOVERAGE (HINN)

Overview

Hospitals issue a Hospital-Issued Notice of Noncoverage (HINN) prior to admission, at admission, or at any point during an inpatient stay if they determine the beneficiary's care is not covered because it is:

- Medically unnecessary
- Not delivered in the most appropriate setting
- Custodial in nature

The four HINNs hospitals issue are:

1. HINN 1: Pre-admission/Admission HINN. Used prior to admission to notify the beneficiary/patient an entirely noncovered stay.

2. HINN 10: Notice of Hospital Requested Review (HRR). Used for Medicare Fee for Service (FFS) and Medicare Advantage Program (Part C) beneficiaries when they request a Quality Improvement Organization (QIO) review of a discharge decision without physician agreement.

3. HINN 11: Used for noncovered items and services during an otherwise covered stay.

4. HINN 12: Should be used in association with the Hospital Discharge Appeal Notices to inform beneficiaries of their potential financial liability for a noncovered continued stay.

For each HINN notification type, the notifier completes the date of notice delivery and beneficiary/patient information (name, patient identifier). Do not use the patient's Medicare number or social security number on this form.

It is the notifier's duty to provide the information required for completion. Explanations may be required, such as why the hospital stay has been deemed no longer necessary for the patient or is no longer covered according to the Medicare guidelines. Best practice is to provide a description for these sections in full sentences and in plain, easy to understand language to illustrate how the patient's condition does not meet the guidelines for admission or ongoing inpatient care.

QIO contact information must be completed on these notices to give beneficiaries the opportunity to discuss and/or appeal the decision. The contact information must be legible, complete, and accurate.

The following are examples of the different HINN notifications and their specific uses:

HINN 1 Preadmission/Admission HINN: the hospital may issue a preadmission/admission HINN when the hospital has determined at the time of preadmission or admission that a beneficiary's stay will be a non-covered stay.

HINN 10 Hospital Requested Review (HRR): When a hospital determines that a beneficiary no longer requires an acute level of inpatient care, but the attending physician does not agree, the hospital may request a QIO review of the medical record known as a hospital requested review (HRR). Hospitals must notify the beneficiary the review has been requested. The QIO review of the hospital's determination considers whether or not continued inpatient care is needed (42 CFR (b)(1), effective July 1, 2005).

HINN 11 is used for non-covered items or services provided during an otherwise covered inpatient stay. The notice may be used to hold beneficiaries liable for certain non-covered services. The item or service at issue must be a diagnostic or therapeutic service excluded from Medicare coverage as medically unnecessary and the beneficiary must require continued inpatient hospital care.

Ensure the Patient Financial Responsibility section is completed as fully and accurately as possible to give the beneficiary the opportunity to make an informed decision on their plan of care and consider potential out of pocket expenses.

HINN 12 is a liability notice to be used in association with the Hospital Discharge Appeal Notices to inform beneficiaries of their potential liability for a non-covered continued stay after the appeal is completed or the time frame for requesting an expedited review is past. The compliance with this notice does not fall under the review authority of the QIO.

This notice requires a date of expected non-coverage, rationale for potential non-coverage, and approximate patient financial responsibility. Consult your case management department leader for the facility specific estimated total or daily care costs.

References

Centers for Medicare and Medicaid. (2018). Hospital Issued Notices of Non Coverage.

Centers for Medicare and Medicaid. (2020). Conditions of Participation. 42 CFR (b).

Resources

Hospital Issued Notices of Non Coverage Forms and Instructions https://www.cms.gov/Medicare/Medicare-General-Information/BNI/HINNs

DETAILED NOTICE OF DISCHARGE (DND)

Overview

A Detailed Notice of Discharge (DND) is given only if a beneficiary requests an appeal. The DND explains the specific reasons for the discharge. A hospital or Medicare health plan must deliver a completed copy of this notice to beneficiaries/enrollees upon notice from the QIO the beneficiary/enrollee has appealed a discharge from an inpatient hospital stay. The DND must be provided no later than noon of the day after the QIO's notification.

The notifier completes the date of notice delivery, beneficiary/patient information (name, patient identifier). Do not use the patient's Medicare number or social security number on this form.

- Section 1 communicates the facts used to make this decision for discharge. The information must be patient-specific and fully describes the patient's current condition, progress and level of function in full sentences, using plain, easy to understand language.

- Section 2 provides a detailed explanation of why the medical inpatient services are no longer covered. Again, the information provided must be detailed and patient specific about why the hospital stay is no longer necessary for the patient or is no longer covered according to the Medicare guidelines. Best practice will describe in full sentences and in plain, easy to understand language how the patient's condition does not meet the guidelines for ongoing inpatient care.

- Section 3 is used for only beneficiaries of Medicare health plans and is used to communicate the plan specific information (policy, provision or stated rationale) related to the determination on non-coverage. As previously noted, the information should be communicated in full sentences of plain, easy to understand language that describe how the services are no longer covered and how the patient's condition specifically does not meet the guidelines or criteria. These forms may be sent to the hospital CM by the Medicare health plan with a request to deliver to the patient in compliance with the Medicare rules.

References

Centers for Medicare and Medicaid. (2018). Fee for Service, Detailed Notice of Discharge.

Resources

Details Notice of Discharge Forms and Instructions https://www.cms.gov/Medicare/Appeals-and-Grievances/MMCAG/Notices-and-Forms

OTHER MEDICARE COMPLIANCE CONSIDERATIONS

Medicare Compliance Consideration are a major focus in running an acute care case management department. I have asked Anna Rheka Winkowski and Jared Johnson to partner with me on these and other topics throughout this book.

MEDICARE POST-ACUTE PATIENT CHOICE

Anna Rheka Winkowski MSN RN CCM ACM-RN

Under 42 CFR § 482.43 Condition of Participation: Discharge Planning, hospitals must focus on the patient's treatment goals and preferences and include the patient and their caregiver in planning their discharge,

> the hospital must include in the discharge plan a list of home health agencies (HHA) or Skilled Nursing Facilities (SNF) that are available to the patient, that are participating in the Medicare program and that serve the geographic area (as defined by HHA) in which the patient resides, or in the case of SNF, in the geographic area requested by the patient (CMS, 2013).

In case management, we always say discharge planning starts on day one and must be constantly re-evaluated during the patient's course of hospital stay. The patient who was independent at the beginning of the hospital stay may be too weak to return home alone and will need some rehabilitation services at a SNF. Similarly, the patient who initially did not have any needs may now require home health services for wound care or physical therapy.

CMs must ensure that patients requiring post-acute services provided the necessary information to be able to select a HHA or SNF of their choice. That does not sound difficult to do, right? But hold on! While the patient can choose post-acute services, your responsibility as a CM is to make sure the patient is making an informed decision when making their selection. How do you do that?

Post-Acute Care Resource List

Before the CM even presents the patient or their caregiver with a list of providers, there are several things to consider. First, the CM must know the patient's payor source(s). Managed Care Organizations have a list of providers within their network the patients choose from. For Medicare patients, providers must be Medicare certified in order to be part of the post-acute provider resource list. Why is this important? If the patient or their caregiver chooses a provider that is not within their network or is not Medicare certified, the post-acute provider may decline the referral—creating double work through another referral to a different provider. Referring to a provider out of network can create avoidable discharge delays, leading to increased length of stay and a dissatisfied patient.

Second, consider the provider's scorecard when it comes to quality measures. The CMS website has a search engine embedded to provide quality information on for skilled nursing facilities/nursing homes, home health and hospice providers. (See Resources at the end of this section). This search engines allow for a focused search for services and provide the overall rating based on the service provider's performance in the health inspections, staffing, and quality of care measures.

Click on the quality-of-care measures rating for the facility and you will be treated to the details of their ratings such as the percentage of short-stay residents who were re-hospitalized after a nursing home admission. If you have a patient who is unable to move themselves on their own, you might want to check the facility's ratings on percentage of short-stay residents with pressure injuries that are new or worsened. If you have a patient whose goal is to return home with maximum functional capacity, you might be interested in checking the facility's percentage of short-stay residents who improved their ability to move around on their own. If your patient or their caregiver is interested in how the facility performed during the health inspections, you can find out when they had their last inspection and how many citations they received compared to the average in the nation or the state.

Typically, the attending physician would come into the patient's room and let them know that they are planning to discharge them home with home health services or to a SNF for some rehabilitation. If the patient has a hospitalist as their attending, the patient cannot be steered toward a certain facility. Having the patient's primary care provider as the attending can get a little tricky because they might try to direct the patients to the SNF where they follow their patients or the HHA where they have some type of financial benefits. Most of the time the patient will agree to go to the facility or use the HHA that their physician is affiliated with. However, as a CM, you must ensure the patient is offered choices of which post-acute provider they want to receive their services from.

42 CFR § 482.43 Condition of Participation: Discharge Planning Paragraph C outlines what requirements apply to be in compliance with providing Patient Choice:

1. A list of post-acute providers participating in the Medicare program must be presented to the patient or their caregivers.

2. The list must take into consideration the geographic area where the patient resides.

3. If the patient is enrolled in a managed care plan, a list of in-network providers must be shared with the patient.

4. There must be documentation that a list was presented to the patient and the patient or their caregiver has provided the discharge planner with their choices.

5. The documentation must be placed in the patient's medical records.

6. Information may be physically printed or electronic or technology based. Referrals should be made to the agency/facility following the facility's case management post-acute referral protocol or the agency/facility process to determine whether the agency/facility can service the patient's needs, works with the patient's payer source and has availability to accommodate patient.

Compliance Best Practice

Patient choice should be confirmed through signature/date by the patient or decision-maker, attesting to the information on the document, using "Patient Choice" form or electronic signature capture as available. *See Figure 5.1.*

If you have a physician who consistently directs patients to post-acute providers where he or she has a financial stake, you must let your physician advisor and your case management director know because this costly mistake could compromise your facility's participation in the Medicare and Medicaid program.

In summary, CMS has made it very clear that patients and their caregivers need to be actively involved in their discharge plan. This occurs by presenting them with a list of post-acute providers participating in the Medicare and Medicaid program, informing them of the providers' quality measures and ratings, allowing the patient to choose a post-acute provider, respecting their preferences, and documenting everything in their medical record.

References

Center for Medicare and Medicaid Services. (2013). Conditions of participation for hospitals, discharge planning. https://www.cms.gov/Regulations-and-Guidance/Legislation/CFCsAndCoPs/Hospitals

Resources

Medicare Care Compare https://www.medicare.gov/care-compare

Confirmation of Patient Choice for

Post Hospitalization Service Providers

1. Your physician has recommended the following post hospitalization services to help you
   continue in your care:
   ☐ Home Health
       o Nursing _____
       o Therapy _____
   ☐ Skilled Nursing Facility
   ☐ Hospice
   ☐ Durable Medical Equipment _____

2. You have the right to use the agency of your choice.
   a. If the agency is not covered by your insurance carrier, this will be discussed with you
      and all options will be discussed (alternatives, self pay arrangements)
3. You have received a list of agency providers of the services that have been recommended for
   you.

STATEMENT OF CONFIRMATION

I have agreed with the recommendation of my physician above and have freely chosen the following
agency(s) to provide post hospitalization services for me. I confirm that I received a listing from which to
choose my service provider from.

   ☐ Home Health _____
   ☐ Skilled Nursing Facility _____
   ☐ Hospice _____
   ☐ Durable Medical Equipment _____

_____   _____

Patient/Representative Signature   Date

_____

Representative's Relationship to Patient

Patient ID label

Figure 5.1 Confirmation of Patient Choice form
Information adapted from Centers for Medicare and Medicaid (2019). Form design by author.

MEDICARE TWO MIDNIGHT RULE (2MN RULE)

Background

Through the Recovery Audit program (RAC), CMS found two significant issues:

1. A higher than average error rate in medical necessity inpatient versus outpatient for short stay admissions.

2. A higher usage of "extended observation services," which led to confusion and significant financial impact for Medicare beneficiaries specifically related to SNF transitions. The Medicare "3 Day Stay" Rule for patients to become eligible for Medicare coverage of their resulting SNF stay uses only inpatient status days to "count" toward the three days. For example, a patient in observation status for three days would not be eligible for Medicare coverage of the SNF stay.

The Two Midnight Rule

As of October 1, 2013, it was determined that:

> Inpatient admissions would be acceptable if the admitting physician had an expectation the patient's care would require being in the hospital through "2 midnights". The medical record documentation must support that expectation. Admissions that were not expected to require "2 midnights" would not be generally approved for inpatient payment. 412.3 (e)(1), Final Rule p 1897 states that "inpatient admissions are 'generally appropriate' for Medicare Part A payment when a physician expects that a patient will need hospital care that crosses two midnights" (Center for Medicare and Medicaid, 2015).

Exceptions to the "Two Midnight Rule":

- Surgeries currently defined as "inpatient only" per the CMS published on the Inpatient Only List

- Patients who expire before two midnights have elapsed

- Patients who choose to leave "Against Medical Advice"

- Patients who elect to start Hospice care

- Patients who have unplanned mechanical ventilation started

- Patients transferred TO another acute care facility

- Patients transferred IN from another acute care facility

Center for Medicare and Medicaid (2015)

Medical necessity remains a critical factor in making the decision to admit a patient as an inpatient. The decision to admit is a complex medical decision that must consider a number of factors including the patient's medical history, co-morbidities, the severity of signs and symptoms, current medical needs, and the risk of an adverse event. All of these factors are considered together to inform a physician's length of stay (LOS) expectation (Center for Medicare and Medicaid, 2015).

Best Practices

- The physician should admit the patient as an inpatient as soon as he or she can reasonably predict the patient will need to remain in the hospital for two midnights or more.
- The physician should not wait until the patient's hospital stay crosses two midnights to write the admission order.
- The clock for the two midnight benchmark starts when the beneficiary begins receiving hospital services, whether inpatient or outpatient.
    - If the patient is kept longer in the hospital because certain care is not readily available (i.e. services not available over the weekend), such delays in the provision of medically necessary care are to be excluded when determining whether the two midnight benchmark has been met.
    - In cases of actual LOS being less than two midnights due to an exception (see exception list) or the rare occurrence where the patient improves more rapidly than the physician expects, inpatient status would still be applicable and conversion to observation status should not be completed.
        - In cases of unexpected improvement, this should be clearly documented in the medical record by the physician.
    - If the physician is uncertain whether the care will extend across two midnights, then the patient may be treated in observation status for the initial day until there is a clear expectation of care crossing the second midnight.
- Admission orders must contain specific wording and phrasing to provide clarity to the admission status (Locke & Hu, 2019).
    - "Admit to Inpatient"
        - "admit to ICU" or "admit to Dr. Smith" should be avoided
        - Proper form: "Admit as inpatient to ICU under Dr. Smith"
    - "Place in Observation Status"
- In addition to the status order, the medical record must state the patient is expected to remain in the hospital for at least two midnights and the reasons for this expectation (referred to as a "certification").
    - As stated in the IPPS rule, "the factors that lead a physician to admit a particular beneficiary based on the physician's clinical expectation are significant clinical

considerations and must be clearly and completely documented in the medical record" (Locke & Hu, 2019).

- The certification does not necessarily need to consist of a separate document.
- The elements of the certification are:
  › Authentication of the practitioner order
  › Reason for inpatient services
  › The estimated time the beneficiary requires or required in the hospital
  › The plans for post-hospital care, if appropriate, and as provided in 42 CFR 424.13

References

Center for Medicare and Medicaid. (2015). Fact sheet: 2 Midnight Rule. October 2015.

Locke, C. and Hu, E. (2019). Medicare's 2 midnight rule: What hospitalists need to know. *The Hospitalist*, February 2019.

Resources

Two Midnight Rule Fact Sheet https://www.cms.gov/newsroom/fact-sheets/fact-sheet-two-midnight-rule-0

TRANSITIONAL PLANNING & THE MEDICARE 3 MIDNIGHT RULE

Jared "Jay" Johnson MSW LMSW CCM

At some point in your career as a CM, you are going to find that you have patients who either need SNF placement, have had it in the past, or are currently receiving services at a SNF. The same can be said for those in smaller rural areas for swing bed (SB). How does one get admitted to one of these facilities? There are more factors to consider beyond skilled nursing needs such as intravenous antibiotics or rehabilitation therapy. The Three Midnight Rule, or more formally referred to as the Three-Day Rule with Medicare, impacts reimbursement. CMS rules state that any Medicare beneficiary must have a qualifying three midnight inpatient stay in an acute care setting within 30 days of the admit date to a SNF or SB (CMS, 2019). Acute care settings could involve an inpatient hospital stay, Intensive Rehabilitation Hospital / Facility (IRF/IRH) stay, or a long-term acute care (LTACH) stay.

Observation Versus Inpatient

A very important detail to explore first would be inpatient versus observation status in a hospital. Whenever a physician writes orders for a patient to be admitted to the hospital, they can order the admittance two different ways. A patient can be admitted as inpatient to the hospital. This is what the general public assumes is happening when they stay overnight in a hospital. Additionally, what could also happen is a physician may elect to have the patient admitted under observation status while they are in the hospital. A physician may elect to determine if a patient needs to be admitted to the hospital, or if they are okay to discharge from the acute care setting. This can be done with an "observation admit". The reason, this is noteworthy, is because, a patient must be inpatient for three midnights, to qualify for SNF services. The inpatient stay does not include time spent in an emergency room, or observation night. For example, if a patient presents to the emergency room Monday, admitted as observation status, then changed to inpatient on Wednesday. The timer for the three midnight would start on Wednesday at the time of the Inpatient order.

Additionally, a physician cannot admit someone to the hospital only to meet a three-midnight rule. The three-midnight inpatient stay must be medically necessary for post-acute SNF/SB services to be ordered or the hospital, SNF, or SB will not be paid by Medicare. If this medical necessity is not met, the patient receives this type of post-acute services and Medicare does not approve payment, the financial burden for the cost of these post-acute services could fall to the patient. Thankfully, many acute care settings have staff that perform Utilization Management (UM) to review patients' medical records, and work as a failsafe to notify physicians if a patient does not need to be inpatient or in the acute care setting at all. However, UM cannot advise or tell a physician what to do. They can only provide information to the physician. Physicians will tell you, both seasoned and new ones, that they never fully understand when an inpatient admit versus an observation admit is appropriate.

Traditional Medicare Versus Medicare Advantage Plans

CM must understand the complicated nuances between inpatient and outpatient status for patients, including differences between tradition Medicare and Medicare Advantage plans. This knowledge is essential for discharge planning and for educating patients and their family members.

Traditional Medicare

Traditional Medicare recipients will require a three-midnight inpatient stay in an acute care setting within a 30-day window prior to the admission to a SNF, or SB. As stated previously, these can consist of a hospital admission, IRF, or LTACH placement. CMs must be mindful of the 30-day rule because it is not uncommon to have a patient discharge from a hospital setting, to return back to the emergency room a few days later. Reasons for returning to the emergency room could include:

- Caregivers were not able to meet needs of patient
- Patient was adamant about being discharged home instead of going to a SNF or SB, and are not safely independent at home
- Patient was nonadherent with prior discharge plan

While these are social reasons for a patient to come back to an emergency room setting, it does not require the patient to be admitted to the hospital. The patient can discharge from the emergency room to a SNF or SB if they have had a three-day inpatient stay in the past 30 days. While it is unfortunate that these situations do happen, they can be managed. The CM can make referrals to any SNF or SB that receives Medicare funding, and the post-acute provider will be able to admit the patient under the medical necessity from the previous admission. As a result, the patient will receive the needed skilled nursing and/or therapy services while the hospital avoids what is called a "social admission."

Examples

- A patient is admitted to an acute care setting as an inpatient. After a patient has been an inpatient for three midnights, they are eligible for a SNF or SB. The time for three midnights starts the moment the provider makes the patient inpatient status. Therefore, if the patient has been medical observation prior to that designation, those nights will not count towards the three midnights.
- A patient was recently discharged from the acute care setting back to their home within the past 30 days. However, during their prior admission they were inpatient for three midnights. While, they were at home, the patient's family decided the patient needs additional therapy. The patient would be eligible for SNF or SB placement.

Medicare Advantage Plans

Medicare Advantage plans appear to be loved and hated by many CMs in many different settings. In situations where a patient needs SNF or SB placement, the three-midnight rule is basically waived. However, the caveat is the SNF will need to be in the Advantage plans network. Medicare Advantage plans are managed policies that still adhere to the Medicare requirements. These plans are generally cheaper to the consumer and offer some benefits that are not covered under traditional Medicare. Understandably, these appear to be more valuable to a consumer at face value.

When a CM is working with a patient in a setting that does have a Medicare Advantage Plan, then they can seek SNF or SB placement as needed. Medicare Advantage plans have their own networks of providers. It is imperative the CM ensures the SNF the patient is interested in, is listed as an in-network provider. Thankfully, this information can be discovered with a Google search.

Example

- A patient presents to the emergency room (ER) after a fall. The patient wants to go to a SNF to get stronger because they noticed reduced endurance during activities of daily living. If the patient has a Medicare Advantage Plan, the CM in the ER can start looking for placement since there is not a three-midnight requirement for Medicare with this patient. Additionally, this could also be completed in a provider's office visit if needed.

Three Day Waiver with Medicare

Just to make things more complex, depending on the area you live at the time of this writing, it's important to consider the Next Generation Accountable Care Organizations (ACO). While Next Generation providers are not spread heavily across the United States, CMs should be aware they exist. If a SNF is part of a Next Generation ACO, then the three-midnight rule with Medicare can be waived. Medicare recipients can benefit from ACO providers, however, the ACO benefits can be a separate discussion.

How do I know if someone is eligible for the SNF 3-Day Waiver?

An individual is eligible for this benefit if they do not already reside in a nursing home or a long-term care facility at the time of admission to a SNF. Additionally, the individual must be medically stable, have a confirmed diagnosis, not require hospital treatment, and have an identified skilled nursing need that cannot be provided on an outpatient basis. If an individual meets all the previously mentioned items and has a doctor who is associated with a Next Generation ACO, then that doctor may admit an individual to a SNF without a three-day hospitalization.

How can a case manager identify an approved SNF?

An approved SNF is one that is participating with a Next Generation ACO and has an overall star rating of three or more under the CMS nursing home comparison. Currently, there are not many facilities that are participating in this program. A CM could simply reach out to a facility that is in question and inquire if they are participating after confirming their star rating using the Medicare Compare tool on CMS website.

Chapter 6:

Quality Considerations

This section again illustrates the depth of the expertise across the care continuum as each of the articles/topics covered in this section are written by experts with experience in the corresponding topics.

QUALITY MANAGEMENT IN PARTNERSHIP WITH CASE MANAGEMENT

Charles White EdD MBA CPHQ

The CMSA Standards of Practice for Case Management (CMSA, 2016) and "The Practice of Hospital Case Management: A White Paper" (CMSA, 2019) provides a sound framework for both clinical and leadership practice. As a professional case manager (CM), carefully review and use the Standards of Practice to expand your oversight and assess the current state of your practice. As you carefully review your job description for expectations and requirements, consider both strengths and opportunities for improvement.

Completing a SWOT (strengths, weaknesses, opportunities, and threats) assessment is a great way to consider your personal strengths and opportunities for improvement, no matter your role. *(See Table 6.1 SWOT Analysis with Sample Considerations.)* It is a great exercise when starting a new position or changing roles. How does your role and the case management department as a whole add value to the organization?

Strengths	Weaknesses
• Competitive Advantages	• Age of Building/Equipment
• Patient Satisfaction	• Financial Resources
• Employee Engagement	• Recruitment & Retention
• Brand Recognition	• Electronic Health Record Limitations
Opportunities	**Threats**
• Supplier Partnership	• New Competitors
• Collaboration with other Departments	• Public Transparency
• Collaboration with External Stakeholders	• Changing Demographics
• Evidence-Based Practice Implementation	• Community Unemployment Rates

Table 6.1 SWOT Analysis with Sample Considerations
Content/layout by author.

After completing your personal assessment, your next step will be to build a 90-Day Plan of Action. CMs are natural leaders, and your personal plan of action provides a strategic roadmap to achieve your personal goals within the department and facility. Within your plan, include both short-term (within 90 days) and long-term goals and objectives that can be linked to the organization. Develop your own individual SMART (specific, measurable, attainable, relevant, time-bound) goals and indicators to monitor your outcomes over time.

Tracking outcomes is a critical strategy in demonstrating the value of case management services. Outcome and process measurement establishes a baseline performance that serves as a starting point for measuring the effectiveness of improvement initiatives over time.   Tracking performance over time also identifies whether our systems, processes, and practices are hardwired for success.

Here are some examples of metrics that can be tracked over time:
- Readmission rates (7, 15, and 30 days; planned and unplanned)
- Avoidable delays
- Overtime
- Patient/client satisfaction
- Employee satisfaction
- Partner/referral satisfaction
- Emergency department returns within 72-hours
- Number of established patient-specific action plans
- Payer pre-certification denials
- Staff turnover
- Social worker response time to high-risk referral or trauma code activation
- Utilization review work queue volume

What other measures could you track to demonstrate the impact of case management?

Once you create your plan of action, share and discuss it with your immediate supervisor. This dialogue is an important step to verify that you are on the right path and obtain buy-in. Review your plan of action at least every 30 days. Take time to evaluate your progress. Review, revise, and add more long-term goals to stretch your individual performance. Celebrate your successes!

Collaborate with Your Organization's Stakeholders

Throughout your education courses, you learned about social systems and systems within the human body (cardiovascular, nervous, skeletal, etc.). Like these examples, organizations function within complex systems that are interactive and cyclical. Communities, regions, and countries are also living systems that respond, react, and adapt to stimuli. We live in a global community of constant change.

Systems Thinking

Case managers are known as "big picture thinkers." Systems thinking is essential when considering how to connect patients with resources post-hospitalization and to continually improve and provide exceptional care delivery. The key to building collaborative, effective, and trusting professional relationships is understanding how you fit into the organization's culture, norms, and values.

Senge (2010) noted that systems thinking is an inherent characteristic of learning and engaged institutions. As CMs, we have an ethical responsibility to provide safe, exceptional care to every individual. Effective assessment requires early identification of opportunities to improve and a plan to change processes and systems to create long-lasting exceptional results.

Develop A Leadership Mindset

It is essential to recognize that your case management "knowledge alone does not include all the attributes that comprise competence, which is a combination of knowledge, skills, and attitude" (Melnyk et al., 2018). As a CM, you will need to collaborate within a more extensive network of interprofessional team members within your organization. You will need to rely on others' guidance to assist you in carrying out your responsibilities. Influential CMs can build trusting relationships with all stakeholders by modeling and reinforcing teamwork, evidence-based practice, and communication.

Communicate

As a CM, you already understand the importance of communication that engages others. Strong communication skills are an essential element of building and sustaining a high-performing team. Engaging other team members and stakeholders through frequent and consistent communication will build stability, transparency, and continuity within the department as a whole.

Be a Financial Steward

Many clinicians find it extremely difficult to bridge clinical practice with business practice. Understanding and embracing your stewardship responsibilities can be a stumbling block. Professional case managers who have a deep understanding of the financial impact of healthcare disparities and reimbursement issues can serve as subject matter experts and guide other interprofessional team members to understand these issues as well.

Expand Your Professional Network

Stay active with professional associations and continue to expand your colleague network. Continuous learning and networking will provide you with the opportunity to access valuable resources and evidence-based practice. Participating in a professional community will help you think outside of the box and consider ways of replicating best practices within your organization.

Learn by Making Mistakes

One of the most incredible learning opportunities is to learn by evaluating your mistakes. Evaluation requires critical thinking and reflection. Having a mentor is a great way to discuss ways of improving your skills and competencies in a safe environment. Mentors also provide you with a different perspective to prompt out-of-the-box thinking.

Take Care of Yourself

Make sure to take time away from your professional responsibilities to recharge and build your resilience. Leading a department will be physically and emotionally draining. You need to schedule time away from work activities to maintain your work and personal life balance.

References

Case Management Society of America (CMSA). (2019). *The Practice of Hospital Case Management: A White Paper.* CMSA: Little Rock, AR.

Case Management Society of America (CMSA). (2016). *CMSA Standards of Practice for Case Management.* CMSA: Little Rock, AR.

Melnyk, B. M., Gallagher, F. L., Zellefrow, C., Tucker, S., Thomas, B., Sinnott, L. T., & Tan, A. (2018). The first U.S. study on nurses' evidence-based practice competencies indicates major deficits that threaten healthcare quality, safety, and patient outcomes. *Worldviews on Evidence-Based Nursing, 15*(1), 16–25.

Senge. (2010). The fifth discipline: The art and practice of the learning organization. New York, NY: Crown Publishing Group.

AVOIDABLE DAYS

Data collection and analysis impact within the healthcare continuum can be demonstrated in examining best practices and practice patterns for potential utilization issues. We all know of the anecdotal "stories from the front" that identify issues and opportunities. However, without the data to support these stories, making the case for a process improvement falls flat.

Reporting avoidable delays helps to identify care gaps and lead process improvement projects. An **Avoidable Delay/Day (AD)** is "any barrier to facilitating effective, efficient, timely, and safe care" (McFolling, 2008). The concept of avoidable delays can be used to "describe barriers that prolong patients' hospital stays when they are medically ready for discharge" (Shelerud & Esden, 2017). It is important to understand how your facility defines an AD. For example, one facility uses the term more broadly to encompass any delay along the continuum of care that creates a delay in execution of the plan of care or discharge. Another facility may define AD as days the patient remains in the hospital while ready for transition to lower levels of care.

Hines and Randall (2010) recommend that professional case managers take the opportunity to review each patient case on a daily basis for instances of ADs. This review will assist in communication to collaborate with care team stakeholders, such as physicians, the case management physician advisor, and ancillary departments to address significant issues in real time and to collect data to support performance improvement initiatives. Through daily rounds and weekly retrospective case reviews, the case management department can more robustly identify, attribute, and report avoidable delays data in an actionable format.

It is also recommended that case management directors and physician advisors have an open dialogue with hospital administration (CEO, COO, CFO) to present ADs data and create actionable plans to resolve systemic issues (Hines & Randall, 2010). These conversations highlight the value of the professional CMs in protecting the organization's financial performance. It's essential for CMs to understand that this type of AD data is valuable to the organization and see improvements based on their documentation of ADs. It is difficult for staff to consider AD documentation a priority if they do not fully understand the value of the tracking or how the data is being used.

> Organizations must actively and consistently use the data collected, which will motivate staff to continue to accurately capture the data. Case managers need consistent education and training on how AD documentation is used and the financial ramifications for lack of documentation (Hines & Randall, 2010).

Being able to categorize delays more efficiently can lead to multiple process improvements including if there is a need to expand lines of services, hours of operation, or provide a return on investment (ROI) analysis to support these initiatives. At one facility, there were 63 Ads in the first six months of the year attributed to lack of cardiology testing on weekends. In these 63 days, the average room and board charges was more than $100,000 in avoidable costs. Additional hospitalized days are associated with higher risks to the patient as discussed in the "Length of Stay" discussion. This information was communicated to senior leadership and immediate action was taken to facilitate weekend cardiology testing.

ADs data can result in better collaboration with post-acute providers for more efficient transitions of care and provide a more effective interface with managed care organizations to expedite determinations. This is accomplished by demonstrating delays in authorization processes and working more effectively across the internal care continuum with multiple disciplines.

Leveraging data could "not only support the process of care delivery, but also promotes better patient outcomes and improvement of health" (Murphy, 2010, p. 205). The CM provides valuable input and insight into driving process improvement. Qualitative data in the form of anecdotal information (or stories) helps to identify potential issues. Quantitative data, as described in the examples given, highlights the severity of the issues and provides insight into potential solutions. Keep telling your stories and back them up with data!

References

Initiatives. (n.d.). Retrieved from Institute for Healthcare Improvement.

Hines, P. & Randall, M. (2010). How do your case managers rate on financial performance? *Healthcare Financial Management, 64*(3), 86–90.

McFolling S. (2008). Data for healthcare improvement—developing and applying avoidable delay tracking. *Collaborative Case Management, 6*(2), 3–12.

Morley, C. (2019). Think case management data doesn't matter? Think again! CMSA Today, March 2019.

Murphy, J. (2010). Nursing informatics: the intersection of nursing, computer and information sciences. *Nursing Economics, 28*(3), pp. 204-207.

Schmidt, B. (2012). The critical importance of good data to improving quality. July / August 2012.

Shelerud, L. & Esden, J. (2017). Case management and the documentation of avoidable days. *Professional Case Management, 22*(2) pp. 64–71.

TRANSFER DRG

History

In the mid-1990s, CMS looked into the transfer of patients along the continuum of care, and more specifically at patients who transitioned from one level of care to another. Prior to Transfer DRGs, the originating acute facility received full payment under the diagnosis related group (DRG) "for providing only part of the necessary care" (Besler, 2020). The stated goal of the Transfer DRG is to prevent CMS from paying for the same care provided for the same patient twice in the same episode. The post-acute transfer (PACT) or Transfer DRG was introduced in the FFY1997 Final Rule and was effective in October 1998.

Several facility types are exempt from the PACT program such as certain sole community hospitals, critical access hospitals and Medicare dependent hospitals.

In 1999, Transfer DRGs started with 10 diagnosis groups. In 2020, there were 278 DRGs. *(See Table 6.2 Number of Transfer DRGs.)* Transfer DRGs are reviewed regularly with diagnosis groups added, deleted, or revised as identified. For example, two DRGs were dropped from the Transfer DRG list in 2020. Transfer DRGs account for 40-50% of Medicare discharges.

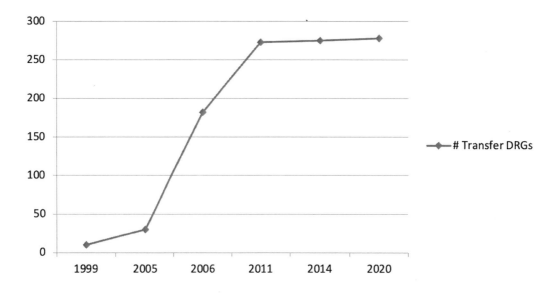

Table 6.2 Number of Transfer DRGs
Data adapted from Wiik, J. (2018). Graph by author.

Definition

CMS pays for Medicare inpatient hospital care under the Acute Care Inpatient Prospective Payment System (IPPS), based on DRGs. When a patient transfers to another provider to continue treatment under certain DRGs (Transfer DRGs), the transferring facility is paid a reduced payment for that care episode.

According to CMS, the Transfer DRG is applicable when:

- The patient's LOS is at least one day less than the geometric mean DRG LOS
- The hospital transfers the patient to another IPPS-covered acute care hospital, or for certain MS-DRG patients, a post-acute setting
- The hospital transfers the patient to a hospital not participating in the Medicare Program
- The hospital transfers the patient to a critical access hospital (CAH)

The Transfer DRG policy includes these post-acute care settings and accompanying discharge disposition codes:

Long-term care hospitals (63)	Rehabilitation facilities (62)	Psychiatric facilities (65)	Skilled Nursing Facilities (03)
Home Health Care (within 3 days after acute stay) (06)	Rehabilitation distinct part units located in an acute care hospital or a CAH (62)	Psychiatric distinct part units located in an acute care hospital or a CAH (65)	Cancer hospitals (05)
Children's hospitals (05)	Hospice care, effective October 1, 2018 (50 or 51)		

Table 6.3 Transfer DRG Codes
Data originated MLN006815 March 2020, p. 14. Table layout by author.

Impact on the Acute Facility (Over/Underpayment)

CMS does audit patient cases, particularly looking at discharge status and discharge dispositions. If CMS finds cases of overpayment due to incorrect discharge disposition reporting, the payment for the entire original bill is recouped. This is a significant financial issue and can be found not just by an audit, but by claim management as well. Wiik (2018) estimates the financial impact can be as much as $1500 per Medicare discharge.

Example: A patient is discharged to home with home health (Disposition Code 06) but the Discharge Disposition is incorrectly documented in the chart/claim as Discharged Home (Disposition Code 01).

1. The facility bills CMS with "01" discharge disposition code.

2. The home health care agency submits their claim for services rendered within three days post-acute discharge. This creates a conflict in claim processing.

3. CMS will recoup the entire payment from the acute care facility.

If the opposite occurred (i.e. the patient was discharged with disposition code 06 instead of 01), it is up to the facility to pursue appropriate and corrected reimbursement. CMS will not reconcile all discharges and claims. It is ultimately the responsibility of the facility to ensure the discharge disposition is correct. *See Discharge Disposition on page 55.*

Best Practices

It is critical for the CMs to ensure the appropriate discharge disposition code is assigned to each patient at discharge. This practice enables the facility to correctly bill and receive the appropriate reimbursement for the patient's care.

References

Besler Consultants. (2015). The history and impact of the Transfer DRG payments.

Centers for Medicare and Medicaid. (2020). Acute care hospital inpatient prospective payment system. MLN Booklet, p. 14.

Wiik, J. (2018). Think you are covered with Transfer DRGs? Think again. December 2018.

READMISSIONS

Since 2009, there has been a focus on readmission reduction and prevention in acute care facilities. Potentially preventable readmissions have been related to failed or ineffective discharge planning especially for patients with chronic diseases such as congestive heart failure (CHF) and chronic obstructive pulmonary disease (COPD). Chronic condition management is a major factor in rising health-care costs. The extensive costs per hospital admission associated with CHF and COPD (to include care, medication, and therapy) represents a major financial liability to health care systems and is considered a significant factor for the issue of unplanned, avoidable readmissions.

The factors driving the need to reduce readmissions include cost containment, achievement of performance initiatives, penalty avoidance, improvement of quality indicators, and high quality patient experiences. National awareness of adverse medical outcomes occurring within care settings continues to rise through quality data reporting, patient satisfaction reports, and a dedication to healthcare transparency. The expanding evidence base points to comparable problems occurring during the transitions between care settings. As case management facilitates and oversees the discharge process, there is a key opportunity to develop interventions to improve the quality of patient transitions from acute care to community with a goal of reducing readmissions.

CMs are in an optimal position to spearhead change in the arena of readmissions. They are adept at care coordination and accessing resources for post-acute care. With an eye to the revenue cycle, they can make an impact by helping the facility to avoid the potential financial ramifications associated with readmissions, improve patient's outcomes, and achieve the patient's goals to remain in their own environment, leading to improved patient satisfaction.

Description and Significance

A readmission is defined as an admission to an acute care hospital within 30 days of discharge from an acute care hospital. The readmission can be related or unrelated to the reason for the initial admission and does not have an impact on the potential for penalties (all cause). Readmissions may also be planned or unplanned and are excluded from readmission penalties. The initial admission which starts the clock (or calendar) on the readmission timeframe is referred to as the index admission (Centers for Medicare and Medicaid, 2020).

According to data from the Center for Medicare and Medicaid Services (CMS), each year, roughly two million patients are readmitted, costing Medicare $27 billion, of which $17 billion is spent on readmissions that could be classified as potentially avoidable. The Med PAC preliminary analysis on readmission trends found the frequency of Medicare patients being readmitted within 30 days of discharge dropped from 16.7% in 2010 to 15.7% in 2017. In 2012, CMS predicted the population of people diagnosed with chronic medical conditions will rise to 125 million by the year 2020 (Center for Medicare and Medicaid Services, 2012). The current trajectory of increase in chronic condition management patients will lead to increased spending at a time when the Medicare program itself appears to be in financial trouble.

Points to Ponder: Impact of Readmissions

- 86% of current healthcare spending is related to chronic conditions
- $1.7 trillion spent on 5% of patients associated with social determinants of health (SDoH)
- $35 million in excess care costs
- $10 billion in illness related lost productivity
- $200 billion related to premature deaths
- $26 billion on readmissions

Information adapted from Institute for Health Improvement Readmissions (2021).

To demonstrate the impact, a CHF patient's 30-day readmission rates are reported as high as 34% and the cost of managing CHF in the United States is estimated to be at least $10 billion per year. It is estimated that currently there are 12.7 million people diagnosed with COPD. The 30-day COPD readmission rates are reported to be 27% nationwide with estimated annual associated costs of $11.9 billion with an average annual cost per beneficiary of $9,545 (Center for Medicare and Medicaid Services, 2020).

Readmission reduction programs have been recommended for implementation. Acute care hospitals have been facing yearly penalties based on readmission rates since the 2012 target date discussed in the original Med PAC report. In a review of 2004 Medicare claims data, Med PAC reported that readmissions accounted for almost 10% of all Medicare expenditures. $17.4 million in spending was attributed to unplanned hospital readmissions and $12 million of that figure were traced to what were identified as preventable readmissions (Medpac, 2007).

Readmission reduction is included in the Patient Protection and Affordable Care Act (PPACA), providing for both penalties and incentives for failure or success in reducing potentially preventable readmissions. Effective October 1, 2012, under Section 3025 of the Affordable Care Act, the establishment of the Hospital Readmissions Reduction Program requires the CMS to reduce payments to participating hospitals with excess readmissions (Center for Medicare and Medicaid, 2020).

Quality initiatives such as The Joint Commission on Accreditation of Healthcare Organizations (TJC) and the National Quality Forum's increased focus on medication reconciliation, discharge planning process and examination of performance measures for post-hospitalization care coordination are examples of endeavors to improve the transitions of care process. Additionally, the Institute of Medicine has advocated for pay for performance measures to motivate healthcare providers to improve patient care coordination across settings. The result is a focus on transitional care, patient satisfaction, and an emphasis on overall quality of care.

The guidelines rolled out by Medicare in 2010 (confirmed by the PPACA in 2012), states readmissions within a 30-day period are reviewed very closely and, in some instances, will not be reimbursed (Centers for Medicare and Medicaid Services, 2020). Facilities with significant readmission rates for certain target diagnoses also run the risk of further financial penalties being imposed for up to 3% of the total Medicare reimbursements for the facility. The financial risk is two-fold; episodic (each readmission after the index admission is at risk of not being reimbursed) and overall penalty (based on percentage of readmissions and measured increase or decrease of readmissions year over year). *See Case Study 6.1.*

The case study reflects an index admission, two (2) thirty day readmission events (no payment), and a potential for higher than average readmission penalty at the end of the year. Additionally, we can use this example to identify gaps in care, extra-medical patient needs that impacted his readmissions, and problem solve for this patient to avoid future readmissions.

Readmission reduction has been identified as a patient safety goal by the Institute for Healthcare Improvement and the Agency for Healthcare Research and Quality (AHRQ). Additionally, the fiscal impact of failing to avoid readmissions, when possible, can lead to a so-called "reputational penalty." Readmissions and penalty data are publicly reported and are figured into the facility's star rating, which can impact the public's perception of the quality of care provided. The emphasis on readmission prevention and the discharge process continues to build momentum with the potential of new diagnoses added each year to Medicare's list. The shift to value-based models and the inclusion of readmission data matters in the discussion of quality of care.

According to the Institute for Health Improvement (2021), current research has demonstrated the rate of readmissions can be reduced by improving discharge planning and care coordination between all levels of the care continuum, concurrent with providing increased opportunities for patient coaching, education, and support for self-management. To decrease readmissions and improve the quality of care, it is suggested to implement an intervention from time of admission through the immediate 30-day post-acute period.

There is no "one-size-fits-all" solution for readmission reduction. Know your population, assess their needs, and make plans to address the issues. Keep in mind that current research notes that only 20% of an individual's health is tied to clinical care, which includes access to and the quality of health care services. 80% of an individual's health is tied to their physical environment, social determinants – where you live, work and play – and behavioral factors including exercise or smoking (Institute for Health Improvement, 2021). The readmission reduction solution a facility chooses to pursue should take these factors into consideration. Preventing readmissions ensures quality of care, reduces costs, protects the facility's financial viability, and improves patient satisfaction.

Case Study 6.1

James is a 68-year-old man who lives at home with his wife of 48 years, Martha. He was admitted to the hospital with shortness of breath and was diagnosed with pneumonia and underlying onset of heart failure. He and Martha were provided with instructions about new medications and a special diet before discharge. James was asked to follow up with his physician in the office in two weeks. A few days after returning home, Martha reminded James to schedule his visit to the physician's office, but James had difficulty reaching the scheduler. Finally, he was able to set up a visit for three weeks later.

James didn't mention to Martha that he took the three day supply of Lasix the hospital sent home with him, but never filled his prescription. He felt well again and thought the expense was unnecessary. When he noticed swelling in his legs, he didn't want to bother the busy doctor and dreaded the ordeal of calling the office again.

After 11 days, James was readmitted to the hospital with increased shortness of breath, marked edema of his lower legs, a weight gain of 25 pounds, and mildly elevated brain natriuretic peptide (BNP)—a marker of cardiac insufficiency. His hospital stay went well, but James' stress level was high, his blood pressure was elevated, and another drug was added to his medication regimen.

While James was in the hospital, Martha was admitted for an emergent surgery. After his discharge, James began eating in fast food restaurants because he was worried about his wife. He juggled visits to Martha's bedside and managed a roofing project on their home. The day Martha came home from the hospital, James was readmitted with exacerbation of heart failure.

References

Askren-Gonzalez, A. & Frater, J. (2012). Case management programs for hospital readmission prevention. *Professional Case Management, 17*(5), 219-226.

Brock, J. (2011). How care coordination affects you. *CMSA Today, 1*(2), 8.

Case Management Society of America. (2016). *Standards of practice for case management.* CMSA, Little Rock, AR.

Cavalier, D. & Sickels, L. (2015). The fundamentals of reducing HF readmissions. *Nursing Management, 46*(11), 17-23.

Center for Medicare and Medicaid Services. (2012). *Hospital Readmission Reduction Program.*

Center for Medicare and Medicaid Services. (2020). *Hospital Readmission Reduction Program.*

Harris, S., Lang, B., Percy, R. & Patronas, C. (2016). Reducing 30-day readmissions for chronic obstructive pulmonary disease. *MEDSURG Nursing, 25*(6), 403-422.

Huntington, M., Guzman A., Roemen A., Fieldsend J., & Saloum H. (2013). Hospital-to home: A hospital readmission reduction program for congestive heart failure. *South Dakota Medicine, 66*(2), 370-373.

Institute for Health Improvement Readmissions. (2021). *Readmissions.*

Medpac (2007). *Report to Congress: promoting greater efficiency in Medicare.* Retrieved from Medicare Payment Advisory Commission.

Stark, J. R. (2010). How can I reduce my facility's readmission rates? *Case Management Monthly, 5*(2), 4.

Resources

Institute for Health Improvement. http://www.ihi.org/Topics/Readmissions/Pages/default.aspx

DENIALS

Mary Jo McHugh BSN RN ACM-RN & Colleen Morley DNP RN CCM CMAC CMCN ACM-RN

Denials represent a serious risk to a facility's financial health. The average hospital has an operating margin of 2%, so even a low denial rate of 2% can wreak havoc on the facility's ability to provide services, continue operations, and expand services to the community. A 5% denial rate at a moderately sized facility can impact over $8,000,000 in revenue annually. For every 1% increase in the denial rate, that's an additional $1,600,000 annually (Advisory Board, 2014).

What's your denial rate?

While the facility is trying to be reimbursed for services provided, the payer is making every effort to decrease costs on their end as well. According to the Advisory Board, a national organization, two-thirds of denials are recoverable and 90% are preventable. The risk to reimbursement is real and effectively managing the denial process is critical from all levels of cases management (department, leadership and individual CMs). Managing denials includes two parts: denial avoidance and denial/ appeal management.

Denial Avoidance

The best defense is a good offense. The utilization management process in any facility is the Denials Avoidance Roadmap. When you follow the process, you can decrease the potential for denials from the outset. In general, denials can be broken into two subgroups: administrative and medical necessity.

Administrative Denials are defined as denials due to a missing administrative component of the process. Examples of these administrative denials include failure to notify the payer in a timely manner or failure to submit clinical reviews in a timely manner. These should both be NEVER events in the case management process because effective communication across the continuum is the forte of CMs.

- Payer notification: During their review of the case, if the CM notes the payer notification has not been completed, it is the responsibility of the CM to initiate the process to ensure the notification is completed. This critical first step of the process may refer the case back to the Notification Department or the CM will initiate the notification process. Doing nothing is not an option here.

- Failure to submit clinical reviews: This is definitely NEVER event in case management. Whatever your facility's model, providing clinical reviews to the payers is a vital part of the utilization review process. Ensuring the clinical reviews are sent to and received by the payer is an essential part of the workflow.

Medical necessity is defined by Medicare as "services or supplies that are needed to diagnose or treat your medical condition and that meet accepted standards of medical practice."

Medical Necessity Denials are adverse decisions made by the payer that the treatment, test, or procedure requested is not medically necessary to treat the patient. This medical necessity can be for level of care (inpatient versus observation or outpatient), treatment, test, or procedure altogether for that particular patient related to their documented conditions and presentation. *See Medical Necessity on page 57.*

Understanding the payer's rules (which criteria sets they use and abiding by their documentation requests) can help ameliorate the medical necessity denial. For example, if the payer is asking for a copy of the status order, send it with your review. If they require a full set of patient vital signs for every reviewed day, then provide it. It can be a bit labor intensive on the front end, but it avoids a denial and appeal on the back end (which takes more time and money to complete).

Understanding agreements in the facility's contract with specific payers is an important part of denial avoidance. Make sure you are informed about any facility-payer specific agreements, such as length of stay for observation cases, non-reviewable diagnoses, etc. Working with the providers and the coding department can ensure a complete picture of the patient is presented to the payer.

Denial Management

The purpose of a denial management process is to investigate denied claims, uncover trends, and appeal the denial appropriately as per the appeals process in the provider contract. Denial management can feel like the song that never ends with steps of reconsideration, first appeal, second appeal etc. However, you need to keep the process going until its conclusion, which can be long and tedious.

So, the case has been denied...now what?! An estimated 65% of denied claims are never resubmitted or appealed. That is a lot of money left on the table! The first rule of Denial Fight Club is to appeal everything that is appealable. The best strategy is to take advantage of all of the steps of the appeal process available to you (Relias, 2018).

1. **Reconsideration**
   Submission of additional clinical information to the payer that may help support the medical necessity of the case.

2. **Peer to Peer (P2P)**
   A conversation between the attending physician and the payer medical director to discuss the clinical aspects and details of the case. This can be extremely useful in cases where the clinical documentation available did not clearly paint the picture of the patient's condition and gives the attending physician an opportunity to "make their case."

3. Formal Appeal

A written request to overturn the denial. Effective appeals letters need to recap the reason the denial was received and the reasons why the denial should be overturned. The key to success is to be complete and have pertinent details of the initial presentation, the clinical progression and impact on the patient, and referencing the criteria used to justify the admission throughout.

There can be several different types or levels of appeal, depending on the payer. Some examples include:

Expedited: if the patient is still admitted to the facility, an expedited appeal can be requested. These determinations are usually available within 72 hours of initial appeal request.

Standard: the patient is usually discharged at the time a standard appeal is processed. The timeframe for submission must be adhered to and the submission needs to include a formal appeal letter discussed previously and possibly, submission of medical records to support the appeal.

Medicare Denials/Recovery Audit Contractor (RAC) Denials

These denials are retrospective denials with the aim of recouping costs for the Medicare Trust Fund.

According to Fierce Healthcare (2018), medical necessity level of care remains the top reason for these denials and subsequent repayments by facilities. It's not the medical care was unnecessary, just that it took place in the wrong setting (INP vs OBS/OP). The good news is the appeal success rate for these denials has been reported as high as 74%. The bad news is that it costs facilities on average of $25,000 annually to manage this process and in some instances up to $100,000.

Medicare Appeals for Recovery Audit Contractor denials have five levels of appeal in order:
1. Redetermination
2. Reconsideration by Independent Contractor
3. Decision by Office of Medicare Hearings and Appeals
4. Review by Medicare Appeals Council
5. Judicial Review in Federal District Court (also referred to Administrative Law Judge or ALJ)

References

Advisory Board. (2014). An ounce of prevention pays off: 90% of denials are preventable.

Arias, P. (2009). Prevent denials and win appeals. HCPro.

Daniels, S. (1999). Using hospital-based case management to reduce payer denials. Healthcare Financial Management, May 1999.

Fierce Healthcare. (2018). Success in proactive denials management and prevention.

Phillips, T. (2017). Ten steps to reduce denials, win more appeals and improve hospital performance. *CMSA Today*, Issue 2, 2017.

Relias. (2018). When managing denials, the best defense is a good offense.

Chapter 7:

Special Topics

As mentioned throughout this book, I am honored to have the input and expertise of subject matter experts. This section's topics of Patient Teaching/Education, the Value of Professional Organizations, and Professionalism in Case Management have been contributed by some esteemed members of our case management community.

SOCIAL DETERMINANTS OF HEALTH (SDoH)

Definition

Social determinants of health (SDoH) can be defined as access to life-enhancing resources (such as food supply, housing, economics, social relationships, transportation, education, health care) whose distribution across populations effectively determines length and quality of life.

Education	Racism/	Employment
Access to health care	Discrimination	Income/Poverty
Environment	Transportation	Housing
Insurance Coverage	Access to Resources	Segregation

Statistics

Only 20% of an individual's health is tied to clinical care, which includes access to and quality of health care services. 80% of an individual's health is tied to their physical environment, social determinants (where you live, work and play), and behavioral factors (including exercise or smoking). More specifically, that 80% can be broken down as follows:

- Roughly 40% is attributed to socio-economic factors
- 10% to physical environment
- 30% to health behaviors

When chronic condition management accounts for 86% of current healthcare spending and the impact of SDoH (80%) is taken into account, the costs to healthcare system can be staggering.

We know the environment where an individual lives and works in addition to non-modifiable health risk factors are inextricably linked. WHERE you live impacts HOW you live. Improving the health of communities cannot be solely focused on individual disease management and treatment, but must address a wide range of factors that shape health status.

SDoH impacts the lives of individuals every day in scenarios such as earning a livable wage, high quality education for children, and access to health promoting situations such as safe parks or grocery stores with fresh produce. Families cannot thrive in unhealthy environments. People living in communities with walking paths and parks are more likely to be active than those who do not have access to outdoor recreational areas. When people have access to healthier foods, they make healthier choices.

All community environments are not created equal when it comes to opportunities for healthy living. Low-income individuals and communities of color are more likely to lack health-promoting infrastructure and resources.

More and more people are recognizing the impacts that chronic diseases such as diabetes and obesity are having on their communities and want to make changes for the health of their families and communities. This movement recognizes that healthy people and healthy places go together. The growing movement for healthy communities—with its push for changes in the physical, economic, social, and service environments—holds great promise.

Life Expectancy Impact

We have established that location matters in concept. Where we live can determine how well we live and is a significant factor of life expectancy. Data from the American Hospital Association (2018) illustrates the range in life expectancy among counties in the United States, from 66 years to 87 years. In some cases, the difference can exceed 20 years. For example, life expectancy rates are lower in southern states than they are in northern states. Even within a single city, along a single street, there can be a dramatic difference in life expectancy.

- In Chicago, babies born a few stops apart on the Chicago Transit Authority's Green Line can face up to a 16-year difference in life expectancy.
- In counties along Route 82 in Mississippi and Alabama, babies can face up to a seven-year difference in life expectancy (American Hospital Association, 2018).

If you are homeless, living in an unsafe or unhealthy conditions, do not have transportation to get to needed medical appointments, or access to food, this greatly impacts your health. Consider the American Hospital Association (2018) data shows that found that children experiencing food insecurity may have two to four times more health problems than children from low-income households who are not food insecure. Adults who are food insecure are also at an increased risk of developing chronic diseases, such as obesity and diabetes. These poor health outcomes contribute to increased rates of readmission and noncompliance, which increases medical costs and risks.

Points to Consider

- How are resources (e.g., food, housing, local businesses, transportation, healthcare services) distributed within your community?
- How does this compare to surrounding communities?

- What are the relationships among social determinants, cultural, and psychological?
- Health starts long before illness in our homes, schools, and jobs.

Healthy People Program

Healthy People 2030 is the fifth edition of Healthy People. It sets goals and objectives to improve the health of Americans through data collection, research, and building on lessons learned from its first four decades. The initiative began in 1979, when Surgeon General Julius Richmond issued a landmark report entitled, Healthy People: The Surgeon General's Report on Health Promotion and Disease Prevention. This report focused on reducing preventable death and injury. It included ambitious, quantifiable objectives to achieve national health promotion and disease prevention goals for the United States within a 10-year period (by 1990). The report was followed in later decades by the release of updated, 10-year Healthy People goals and objectives (Healthy People 2000, Healthy People 2010, Healthy People 2020).

Target Year	Overarching Goals	Number of Topic Areas	Number of Objectives
1990	Decrease overall mortality rate Increase independence in > 65-year-old population	15	226
2000	Increase healthy life span. Reduce health disparities. Increase access to preventive care services for all	22	312
2010	Increase quality and longevity of healthy life. Eliminate health disparities.	28	
2020	High quality longer lives without preventable disease. Achieve health equity by eliminating disparities. Create health social and physical environments. Promote quality of life, healthy development, and behaviors throughout life	42	Over 1200

Table 7.1 Healthy People Program
Data adapted from Healthy People.gov (2020). Table layout by author.

Healthy People 2020 Priority Issues Related to SDoH

Neighborhood/Built Environment

- Quality of housing
- Crime and violence
- Environmental conditions
- Access to healthy foods

Education

- High school graduation rates
- Enrollment in higher education
- Early childhood education/development
- Language/literacy

Economic Stability

- Poverty
- Employment
- Housing stability
- Food insecurity

Health and Health Care

- Access to health services
- Access to primary care
- Health literacy

Social and Community Context

- Social cohesion
- Perceptions of discrimination and equity
- Civic participation
- Incarceration/institutionalization

Adapted from Healthy People.gov (2020).

Healthy People 2030 Goals (HealthyPeople.gov, 2020)

- Attain healthy, thriving lives, and well-being, free of preventable disease, disability, injury and premature death.

- Eliminate health disparities, achieve health equity, and attain health literacy to improve the health and well-being of all.

- Create social, physical, and economic environments that promote attaining full potential for health and well-being for all.

- Promote healthy development, healthy behaviors and well-being across all life stages.

- Engage leadership, key constituents, and the public across multiple sectors to take action and design policies that improve the health and well-being of all.

Real Life Examples of SDoH in Action

The EveryONE Project

- Developed by American Academy of Family Physicians (2016), asks the question "Why treat people and send them back to the conditions that made them sick in the first place?"

- Assessment toolkit developed

Coordinating Transitions (CT), reported by Morrison (2017).

- Integrated SDoH into practice workflow using existing electronic medical record (EMR)/Health Information Exchange (HIE) and electronic data

- Includes a Patient Centered Assessment Method (PCAM) that scores and standardizes identification of social problems that place an individual at risk for hospitalization

- Contributed to decreased emergency department (ED) use (over 700 visits) and hospital admission rates (over 80 admissions) over 2-year study period

Transforming Complex Care (TCC) by Thomas-Henkel, C. & Schulamn, M. (2017)

- Multistate initiative under Robert Wood Johnson grant

- Uses "PRAPARE" tool or home-grown screening tool

- Focus on data collection, electronic implementation

Advocate ACO Nutrition Program, reported by Morrison (2017).

- Two initiatives

- High risk patients (malnutrition) receive oral nutritional supplement within two days of admission

- Enrolled in post-acute program: nutrition education, follow up calls, coupons and oral nutritional supplementation

- Total savings $4.8 million, decreased readmission rate

West Suburban Medical Center "Eat & Be Well Medical Pantry" (Levin, 2018)

- Collaboration with Temple Jeremiah, Great Chicago Food Depository
- Patients receive a prescription from the pantry, operated once a week
- Lean meats, fresh produce
- Follow up with a physician in six weeks to renew prescription

ProMedica, reported by Koh et al, 2020

- 332 sites of care, 4.7 million encounters, 13 hospitals and 323,000 lives
- Toledo, OH project: "Food Pharmacy"
- Healthcare provider writes a referral and identified patients visit and pick up supplemental health food supply
- 57,224 patients screened in 2016 and 2243 screened positive, 1100 became food pharmacy clients
- ED usage dropped 3%, readmission rates dropped 53%, and primary care visits increased by 4%

Multisite Transportation Projects (reported by Koh et al, 2020)

- Team with Uber/Lyft (MedStar, Denver Health)
- Mobile treatment facilities (Calvert Health, MD)

University of Illinois Housing Project (Brown, et al, 2018)

- Targeted 200 chronically homeless individuals in the highest category for patient/healthcare cost
- Partnered with Center for Housing and Health to create "Better Health Through Housing" in 2015. This project included identification and assessment of these patients when they present to the ED.
- Criteria: Continually homeless for a year or more or more than four episodes of homelessness within a three year period.
- Patients were moved to the "bridge unit" (transitional housing) and work with CM for long term housing solutions
- Outcomes: ED use decreased by 35%, increased clinic use, healthcare costs dropped 42% initially and most recent results show 61% reduction

Mount Sinai Hospital/Sinai Health Urban Health Institute CHW Program (Jay, et al, 2021)

- Use of Community Health Workers for post-acute home visits
- Started with asthma in 2011, CHW sent to identify triggers to exacerbations (environmental, behavioral, etc.)
- In the first year reduced asthma ED visits by 73% and hospitalization by 75%

Case Study 7.1

Meet William. William came to our hospital with an infected wound on this foot, but in truth, his troubles were greater than what was presented. When I first met William, he was an affable, but guarded patient. He was willing to answer questions, but only to a certain point, when he started to be evasive. The next time I went to speak with him, he was in full blown withdrawal from his heroin addiction.

During his admission, his discharge concerns continue to mount. He was homeless, uninsured, without an income, without family or other social supports, and without a primary care physician all of these issues making it difficult to obtain the medical care he needed to heal his infected foot. He needed antibiotics, a substance abuse program, a clean place to change his dressings, follow up at wound care clinic, a primary care physician, and lastly, transportation to all his appointments.

What Can You Do for William?
- Identify issues
- Prioritize issue
- Solve issues

After meeting with him a few times, William was agreeable to try a Suboxone program for his heroin use issues. One of the hospital's affiliated clinics had such a program and could enroll him in it. His hospital physician was also on staff with the same clinic and was willing to continue to see William as an outpatient even with his current financial status.

Financial counselors were contacted and they, with William, began his application for Medicaid. We were also able to find him temporary, but transitional, shelter at a facility that worked with the homeless who needed medical care. William now had a place to live for a while, where he could care for his foot in clean environment. A call to the wound care clinic was made and after some advocating, they were willing to see William, knowing his insurance had not been yet approved. They would monitor the healing of his foot ulcer. The hospital's medication program was able to provide the patient with his antibiotics and the nursing floor at discharge provided him with extra dressing changes until he could go to the wound care clinic. The hospital provided bus passes for William to get to all his appointments.

I met with William about two to three times a week to check in with him and to provide the needed bus passes. About four weeks into the situation, I saw William and he stated he was doing well. He was still attending the substance abuse program and remained abstinent. He was continuing with the wound care clinic and his foot was doing much better and was well on the way to being healed. I offered him some more bus passes for transport, but he declined stating he didn't need them. How was he to get to his appointments? He smiled at me stated, I got a job! He had started a new job the previous week and was getting his first paycheck that day. He was grateful for all we had done but didn't want to continue to take what he didn't need. He turned gave me a huge hug and went off to work.

I heard from William about three months later. He was still substance free; the wound was healed, and he was still working. He had found an apartment and was making headway with rebuilding relationships. The stars and planets had aligned, and he was following their path. This is what case managers and social workers do. We give the push in the right direction for others to have their needs fulfilled.

(Used with permission, CMSA Chicago, 2019, E Bergman & C Morley editors. Contributed by E. Walker)

HEALTH LITERACY

Health literacy is defined as the degree to which an individual has the capacity to obtain, process, and understand basic health information and services needed to make appropriate health decisions. Osbourne (2013) goes a step further in defining health literacy as "a shared responsibility between patient (or other recipient of the health communication) and providers (or other "giver" of the health communication)." Bi-directional communication is a MUST. Health literacy differs from basic literacy (or the ability to read) in the concept of processing the information into action.

With health literacy being identified as not only a social determinant of health (SDoH), but as the newest vital sign, "addressing patient health literacy and health confidence is as much a necessity as identifying patient's extra-medical needs and linking with needed services and resources to provide the patient with excellent patient-centered care, promote client self-advocacy and independence in alignment with the CMSA Standards of Practice" (Morley & Walker, 2019).

Current statistics demonstrate that 36% of the population of the U.S. is rated as basic or below basic literacy (reading) level. The health literacy rate is significantly lower than this at 12% (Agency for Healthcare Research and Quality (AHRQ), 2018). Health literacy is considered a SDoH and a key in patient safety that should be assessed and addressed for every patient, every time, in every healthcare encounter. The need to focus on health literacy goes to the core of healthcare. Although the evidence supports that some populations are at higher risk for lower literacy and health literacy rates, anyone can be affected by low health literacy. People who may have been previously able to self-manage may no longer be able to do so. Research on health literacy has shown that patients with poor health literacy are less likely to consistently access preventative care. They are less able to successfully manage when diagnosed with chronic disorders and incur higher healthcare costs, use the emergency department for healthcare more often, and are more frequently readmitted after acute care discharge (AHRQ, 2018).

Wagner's Chronic Care Model seeks to "optimize each healthcare team member's abilities, expertise and willingness to achieve high-quality health outcomes…that are safe, necessary, cost-effective, timely, desired and patient-centered" (Potter & Wilson, 2017, p. 311). Patients engaged in this model study reported higher satisfaction with the healthcare team, their healthcare experience, and increased confidence in managing their chronic conditions. In this era of patient-centered care, the patients and their caregivers are identified as part of the healthcare team. As such, it is vital the information transfer between patient and provider(s) is clear, understood, and actionable by the patient or caregiver. To enhance patient engagement and likelihood of success, it's essential to assess the patient's and caregiver's preferred learning styles and understand how to leverage the roles of the healthcare team to meet those needs.

The professional case manager applies this theory by educating and providing coordination of care, services, and resources in alignment with the patient's needs, provider's recommendations, and benefits available under the patient's payer plan and network. The Standards of Practice for Case Management direct CMs to assume the role of "advocates who help patients understand their current health status, what they can do about it and why those treatments are important… by guiding patients and providing cohesion to other professionals in the health care delivery team, enabling their clients to achieve goals more effectively and efficiently" (Case Management Society of America, 2016, p. 3).

Tips for Case Managers to Address Health Literacy

- Assess every patient, every time you meet with them.
- Don't assume there have been no changes, even day to day
- Use plain language
- Keep away from medical healthcare jargon
- Limit information
- 3-5 key points per encounter, revisit/reinforce
- Be specific, avoid generalizations
- Demonstrate, draw pictures, use models.
- Don't rely on verbal/written communication.
- Repeat, summarize, or restate a different way
- Teach back!
- Confirm the patient and caregiver understood the information you just taught them by asking them to demonstrate or explain what they have learned.
- Be positive, hopeful, and empowering!
- You are their lifeline and cheerleader
- Consider the impacts of health literacy in every intervention, every project

Source: Data in this table adapted from AHRQ (2018).

Unless health literacy is better understood and addressed, it is less likely that there will be an environment created where patients are engaged, empowered, and able to achieve self-care with greater confidence and success. The question we need to ask is "how do we, as healthcare practitioners, engage and empower our patients and their caregivers to be successful in managing complex medical issues combined with the day to day business of living?" Once asked, we need to create sustainable education strategies and opportunities for the 88% of the population who do not have adequate health literacy.

> **Best Practice Resource**
>
> AHRQ Health Literacy Universal Precautions Toolkit
>
> https://www.ahrq.gov/health-literacy/improve/precautions/index.html

References

Agency for Healthcare Research and Quality (2018). AHRQ Health Literacy Universal Precautions Toolkit.

Brock, J. (2011). How care coordination affects you. CMSA Today, 1(2), 8.

Case Management Society of America. (2016). *Standards of practice for case management.* CMSA, Little Rock, AR.

Morley, C. & Walker, E (2019). Health Confidence, Health Literacy & Readmissions. *CMSA Today, 3*(19).

Pomerantz, J., Toney, S. & Hill. Z. (2010). Care coaching: An alternative approach to managing comorbid depression. *Professional Case Management, 15*(3), 137-42.

Potter, M. & Wilson, C. (2017). Applying bureaucratic caring theory and the chronic case model to improve staff and patient self-efficacy. *Nursing Administration, 41*(4), 310-320.

Watson, J. (2006). Caring theory as an ethical guide to administrative and clinical practices. *Nursing Administration, 30*(1), 48-55.

Resources

AHRQ Health Literacy Universal Precautions Toolkit https://www.ahrq.gov/health-literacy/improve/precautions/index.html

IMPLICIT BIAS IN HEALTHCARE

Implicit bias can be defined as unconscious stereotypes that can impact our decision-making process. Everyone has them. How do professional CMs learn to recognize and overcome them in working with our diverse client populations?

Implicit bias "refers to attitudes or stereotypes that affect our understanding, actions, and decisions in an unconscious way, making them difficult to control" (Ruhl, 2020). Implicit has its roots in the hidden attitudes we all have, based on social stereotypes that are activated by our subconscious fast-moving brain. Explicit bias is defined as those biases that we are aware of possessing and then act upon. This is a slower thought process where attitudes are developed over time and with a conscious decision to adopt as our own.

An implicit bias may run opposite to a person's conscious beliefs without them realizing it. "For example, it is possible to express explicit liking of a certain social group or approval of a certain action, while simultaneously being biased against that group or action on an unconscious level" (Ruhl, 2020).

Implicit bias in healthcare can be illustrated with the following types of examples:

1. When the Implicit Association Test (IAT) was administered to participants at an obesity conference, the responses implicitly associated obese people with negative cultural stereotypes, such as "bad, stupid, lazy and worthless" (Schwartz et al., 2003).

2. A child presented with respiratory issues that had so far defied explanation. The team of physicians were agonizing over the patient's x-rays, puzzled because a diagnosis could not be agreed upon. Another physician just passing through the workroom looked at the x-rays and immediately said, "cystic fibrosis." The team has been tripped up by the patient's race, which was black, and never considered cystic fibrosis as a possibility, categorizing it as a "white disease" (The Joint Commission, 2016).

It is important to understand that implicit biases can become an explicit bias. To do this, you must become purposefully aware of the prejudices and beliefs you possess and consciously decide to act on them.

The human brain tends to generalize and seek out patterns to create "mental shortcuts" or "decision efficiencies" to speed up decision making in a complicated world. These mental shortcuts aid in decision making ("rules of thumb") and make it easier for people to process the overwhelming stimulus we receive every minute of every day. Don't discount the impact of social or cultural influences from the individual experience to cultural group, societal perceptions, or media depictions on the development of implicit bias.

Healthcare Impact

Disparities in healthcare for diverse populations continue, despite many years of focus under the Healthy People 1990-2020 agendas. Before we look at the external contributors, we must, as healthcare providers, look within and do a "self-check" on our own implicit biases and the effect they may have on our delivery of care. Indeed, clinician bias has been identified as a contributing factor to health care inequalities.

Patient perception of provider bias can have adverse effects on patient experience, engagement, trust in the healthcare provider and by extension, the healthcare system. CMSA Standards of Practice and Code of Professional Conduct speak to being advocates for our patients to ensure that we act in their interests, respect their rights and dignity, maintain objectivity, and act with integrity and fidelity in all aspects of care provided and interactions we have as professional CMs.

Everyone has implicit biases; it's just how the human brain is wired to work. We need to recognize what they are for each of us, as individuals, and "do the work" to ensure these "mental shortcuts" do not impact the care we give to our patients, promote healthcare equity, and reduce the healthcare disparities in the system. To help you identify your own implicit biases, Harvard University has developed "Project Implicit," a series of self-administered tests to do a self-assessment on your own understanding of attitudes and stereotypes. The tests cover bias identification in a variety of sub-topics, such as race, weight, gender, transgender, sexuality, culture, and age. Access this project through the link in the Resources list.

References

Blair, I. V., Steiner, J. F., & Havranek, E. P. (2011). Unconscious (implicit) bias and health dis-parities: Where do we go from here? *The Permanente Journal, 15*(2), 71–78.

Centers for Medicare and Medicaid. (2017). Guide to preventing readmissions among racially and ethnically diverse beneficiaries.

Commission for Case Manager Certification. (2015). The Code of Ethics and Professional Conduct for Case Managers, The Commission for Case Manager Certification, Mount Laurel, NJ.

Dovidio, J.F. & Fiske, S.T. (2012). Under the radar: How unexamined biases in decision making processes in clinical interactions can contribute to healthcare disparities. *American Journal of Public Health, 102*(5): 945.

Fink-Samnick, E. (2016). Case Management Ethics 2017: Where Should Your Ethical Compass Point? AAMCN Fall Conference, November 2016.

Fink-Samnick, E. & Muller, L. (2013) Ten steps to navigate ethical, legal challenges in case management.

Harvard University. (n.d) Project Implicit.

Ruhl, C. (2020, July 01). *Implicit or unconscious bias.* Simply Psychology.

Schwartz, M. B., Chambliss, H. O., Brownell, K. D., Blair, S. N., & Billington, C. (2003). Weight bias among health professionals specializing in obesity. *Obesity Research, 11*(9), 1033–1039.

The Joint Commission (2016). Quick Safety 23: Implicit Bias in Healthcare. Issue 23.

Treiger, T. and Fink-Samnick, E. (2015). COLLABORATE® for Professional Case Management: A University Competency-Based Paradigm, 1st Edition, Wolters Kluwer, Philadelphia, PA

Van Ryn, M., Burgess, D.J., et al (2011). The impact of racism on clinician cognition, behavior and clinical decision making. *DuBois Review, 8*(1): 199-218.

Resources

Project Implicit. https://implicit.harvard.edu/implicit/takeatest.html

GUARDIANSHIP: WHAT CASE MANAGERS NEED TO KNOW

Teri Dreher RN iRNPA CCM

Typically in hospitals when case managers encounter someone who has no one to care for them and no resources, the public or state guardian's office is called to evaluate the patient for guardianship. When people have no money or very little money (less than $30,000 in total assets), this is generally the best course of action because the guardianship process can be costly and time consuming. Sometimes counsel for the hospital is consulted and they can usually get into court quickly to initiate guardianship proceedings. Unfortunately, this costs the hospital a lot of money because attorneys are expensive, not to mention how many days it takes to get a court hearing to assign emergency (temporary) guardianship, which only lasts for 60 days.

The temporary guardian can often petition the court to allow placement in a SNF or group home if funds allow. The process can happen in as little as three days if the report and CCP211 document are done on the same day, and an attorney delivers the documentation to the Clerk of Court in the county the respondent lives in. Usually, it takes between 10-14 days to get in front of a probate judge who is able to approve temporary guardianship, and then the guardian can place the patient in a safe environment.

Guardianship Basic Training

- **Who may have a guardian appointed?** A guardian may be appointed to serve as a substitute decision-maker for a person, who for reasons of mental deterioration or cognitive decline, physical incapacity, or developmental disability cannot make or communicate responsible decisions about his/her personal affairs. In cases where a person is exposing him/herself to risk by "gambling, idleness, debauchery, excessive use of intoxicants" and harming himself or his family by these activities, counsel should be sought, because today it is rare for judges to take away rights due to poor life decisions. It is a serious infringement on an individual's rights to take rights away. Only a court can invoke guardianship after a careful review of other less restrictive options.

- **Preliminary Steps:** First, a pre-printed form obtained from the Clerk of Court's office needs to be completed, describing the nature of the respondent (patient's) disability, and how it impacts their ability to function independently. This is called a CCP211 form and can only be signed by a physician, with help from other parties that can state the evidence of the disability. It must say what kind of guardianship is necessary: temporary, limited, or plenary (total) guardianship, and should include as many details as possible. The more thorough the physician's evidence and diagnoses, the better.

- **Attorney representation:** Advice of counsel is highly recommended, either for the family, hospital, or petitioner (person making the request). They ensure deadlines are met and keep us compliant with every tiny rule. Families can petition the court without representation. Frivolous claims due to family dissension are not tolerated well by judges and embarrassing for those who attempt them. A Guardian Ad Litem (GAL) is almost always appointed by the court to represent the best interests of the respondent and goes to see the person in their home, meeting with them often several times to interview the patient about whether he/she agrees to guardianship. If he does not, then the court will appoint an attorney to represent the patient. In private guardianship, guardians of estate, person and all attorney fees generally come out of the patient's estate. Guardianship is very much about protecting the person and their resources.

- **Preparation for Court:** Once a CCP211 form is obtained by the hospital, attorneys prepare an official petition, a Rights notice, a Summons to the respondent (generally delivered by the sheriff), a Notice of Interested Parties, an order, an Oath of Office, obtain a Surety Bond from those who will handle finances (Guardian of Estate), a Statement of Right to Discharge Guardian if need before to alter the original order, and an order for the court to appoint a GAL.

- **Court:** Court is presently being done mostly virtually now during COVID and it is uneventful. You need to be prepared to give accurate testimony. The original temporal guardianship order lasts only 60 days, which gives the Guardian of the Estate (GOE) time to do a search on the respondent's assets. The court generally appoints the temporary guardians at the first hearing and may need one or two extensions before going to the court to ascertain if plenary guardianship is necessary. If so, at that time, we are sworn in and take an oath to abide by all laws and deadlines.

The primary role of the CM in a hospital is to discharge patients to the safest, most appropriate option in the community as quickly as possible, to save money for costly stays after the patient is medically stable to leave. If the patient is medically complex, has no family, and no one willing to assume responsibility for the patient's care, pursuing guardianship may be your only recourse.

"The ultimate moral test of government is the way it treats those who are in the dawn of life, the children; those who are in the twilight of life, the elderly; and those who are in the shadows of life, the sick, the needy, and the handicapped."

— Hubert H. Humphrey

Case Study 7.2

After one of my recent speaking events for hospital CMs, one person who attended my talk on Senior Orphans called to tell me a sad story about a fellow I will call Fred. Fred was a widower, had no children, and the few relatives he once had had long passed away. He was one of those MVPs: multi visit patients. He kept falling at home, getting a couple of weeks of home healthcare, and then being discharged with no one to help him. He refused home care due to the cost and had had multiple referrals to Adult Protective Services (APS), which resulted in no decisions regarding his lack of ability to care for himself.

The CM had taken a special interest in Fred and was frustrated that he was not able to care for himself adequately. She worried the next admission may be more serious. What should be done in this case? I promised to visit and see if we could get my company to sign on, even as a pro bono client. He resolutely refused to sign anything when I met him and told some stories about past "helpers" who had likely financially exploited him. He was wary and warned me not to talk to either of his neighbors, who he had found rummaging through his desk upstairs when uninvited. So, I asked him if we could just come in and check on him every so often and make sure the wound on his leg was properly cared for. He agreed and we worked with Fred for about six weeks uneventfully until his wound was better and he was okay on his own now.

One Saturday morning a few weeks later, I woke up thinking about Fred and decided to pay him a visit myself. I drove down to his home, which he had told us he owned outright and when I knocked on the door, I could see the lock had been damaged and the door swung open. I called out to him, and he answered, "Help! I have fallen and can't get up!" It was just like the commercial on TV. I entered with his permission and saw a sad sight. Fred had fallen in his kitchen on his left hip, and I was afraid he had broken it. I called 911 and assured him we just needed to make sure he had not broken anything. He had been on the floor for most of the night, he said. He was weak, confused, and his clothes were so soiled that I was sure he had not bathed in weeks. His home was in disarray and the whole house was in a terrible state of disrepair, with mold growing over one half of his dining room wall. An upstairs toilet had been leaking and was full of stool.

Though the hospital ED staff would not talk with me as I was not family or in any official capacity, I left and called the hospital CM the next day, enlisting the referring CM's help at their sister hospital to get needed information for the staff to evaluate him for competency. Fred was admitted for a mechanical fall, but his real issue had been decompensation of congestive heart failure, as well as dehydration, malnutrition, and a new NSTEMI. He was quite complex.

After a few days of good care, he was medically stable for discharge. After talking with the hospital, we were able to get Fred transferred to a good rehab facility. A psychiatrist's evaluation made it possible to initiate guardianship proceedings. He is now our ward and is the delight of the SNF where he permanently resides after completing his rehab days. All the staff members absolutely love Fred, and he says he is so happy there; he can't believe he gets to live there. He has gained 17 lbs. so far and is quite the social butterfly. I have it on good authority that Fred has had several residents propose marriage in the past month.

It is stories like Fred's that make me realize that this work is needed and very worthy in today's world. With rising numbers of seniors aging alone in America, I feel it is a social justice issue to protect them, honor them, and care for them as the valuable people that they are. They are part of our rich country's heritage, and in a day when ageism is everywhere, we look, we need to remember to pay it forward, for one day all too soon, we will be there ourselves. Care managers and advocates make such a huge difference to the vulnerable.

ABUSE AND NEGLECT: THE WHO, WHAT, WHY, AND HOW OF REPORTING RISK TO VULNERABLE POPULATIONS

Introduction

Acute care facilities are mandated to help protect vulnerable populations in accordance with local, state, and federal abuse reporting laws. Hospital protocols include assessment, intervention, documentation, and referral of all situations that could be abuse or neglect. All levels of clinical facility staff are educated about the signs, symptoms, and physical indicators of abuse and/or neglect in addition to the reporting requirements for each population. All professional CMs should be educated in identifying and reporting possible victims of assault, abuse and/or neglect per local, state, and federal laws.

Pertinent Definitions from Center on Elder Abuse (2019)

Abuse

Abuse is the direct infliction of, the toleration of or the causation of a substantial risk of:

- Physical, non-accidental injury which causes death, disfigurement, impairment of physical/emotional health or loss/impairment of any bodily function (i.e., burns, failure to thrive)

- Any sexual offense

- Any act which harms any person

This can take many forms, such as:

- Physical: an act that results in bodily harm, injury, impairment or disease, hitting, slapping, striking, sexual coercion/assault, incorrect positioning of the elder, forced feeding, forced medicating, improper use of restraints

- Sexual: any sexual contact with a person who, because of mental illness or dementia, cannot communicate their disapproval of the behavior against them or cannot communicate consent for the activity. Whether or not the contact is significant or minor, if it is sexual in nature and nonconsensual, it is sexual abuse

- Emotional/Psychological: inflicts emotional pain or distress, verbal scolding, harassment, intimidation, threatening punishment or deprivation, isolation

- Financial exploitation: taking control of the resources of another through misrepresentation, coercion or outright theft for their own gain

Neglect

- Abandonment
- Physical: the withholding or denying of nourishment or medically indicated treatment, clothing, or shelter necessary for well-being, failure to provide physical aids or safety precaution
- Psychological: failure to provide social stimulation, leaving someone alone for long periods of time, failing to provide companionship or links to the outside world
- Financial Failure: to use available resources to sustain or restore health and security. Improper level of care when there are resources available to provide the proper level of care, sudden transfer of assets
- In a newborn with evidence of a controlled substance (or related metabolite) in blood or urine (unless medically indicated for the mother or newborn).

Neglect is **not** reliance upon spiritual means through prayer alone for remedial care or the treatment/cure of disease. Examples include a Jehovah's Witness patient refusing blood products or Christian Scientist members refusing medical care.

Population Descriptions

Four population types addressed are:

- Child (age 0-18 yrs.)
- Elder (age 65+ yrs.)
- Domestic abuse (no age defined)
- Vulnerable adult is an individual, 18 years of age or older whose ability to perform the normal activities of daily living or to provide for his or her own care or protection is impaired due to a mental, emotional, long-term physical, or developmental disability or dysfunction, or brain damage, or the infirmities of aging.

Domestic Abuse

Domestic abuse is physical abuse, harassment, intimidation of a dependent or family member, threats, interference with personal liberty or willful deprivation and can include the following:

- Either battering or abusive acts within a family or intimate relationship.
- Physical abuse, harassment, intimidation of a dependent or family member, threats, interference with personal liberty or willful deprivation.
- Domestic violence can take many forms, such as verbal harassment, kicking, choking, fighting and biting.

Mandated Reporter

Mandated reporters are professionals, who, in the ordinary course of their work, and because they have contact with children, disabled persons, senior citizens, and other identified vulnerable populations, are required to report or cause a report to be made, whenever financial, physical, sexual or other types of abuse have been observed or is suspected or when there is evidence of neglect, knowledge of an incident or imminent risk of harm.

Persons not identified as mandated reporters are nevertheless encouraged to report suspected abuse and neglect. Individuals who do report are protected from civil and criminal liability. However, making a false report constitutes a misdemeanor.

Reporting domestic abuse (domestic violence) is voluntary unless there is a serious injury, or it involves a deadly weapon. Familiarize yourself with all pertinent policies, procedures and laws in your practice area.

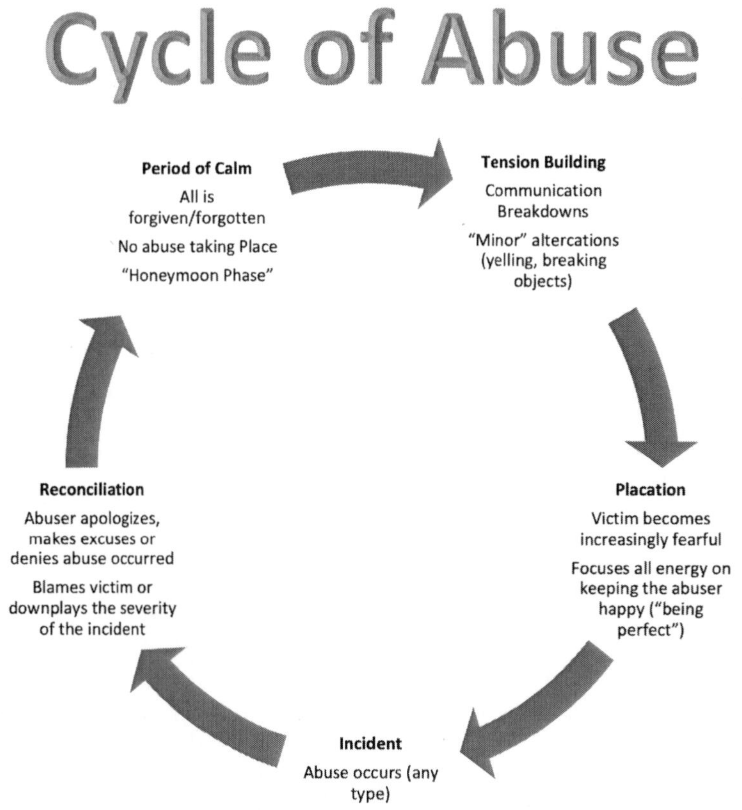

Cycle of Abuse

Period of Calm
All is forgiven/forgotten
No abuse taking Place
"Honeymoon Phase"

Tension Building
Communication Breakdowns
"Minor" altercations (yelling, breaking objects)

Placation
Victim becomes increasingly fearful
Focuses all energy on keeping the abuser happy ("being perfect")

Reconciliation
Abuser apologizes, makes excuses or denies abuse occurred
Blames victim or downplays the severity of the incident

Incident
Abuse occurs (any type)

Chart 7.1 Cycle of Abuse
Adapted from Bullock, et al. (1989). Figure layout by author.

Statistics

Child Abuse

In 2018, the most recent year for which there is national data, an estimated 678,000 children were victims of abuse and neglect. This number represents about 1% of children in the U.S. Sadly, it is assumed that this information is incomplete and the actual number of children abused is under reported. In that same year, an estimated 1,770 children died from abuse and neglect. The youngest children were the most vulnerable. 2.7% of children in the first year of their life had the highest rate of abuse reports parent (National Children's Alliance, 2020).

Neglect is identified as the most common form of abuse, and accounts for about 61% of reports The remaining 39% of reports were made for abuse: 10% for physical abuse and 7% were sexual abuse. More than 15% of kids were reported to suffer two or more forms of abuse. In substantiated child abuse cases, and 78% of children were victimized by a parent (National Children's Alliance, 2020).

Elder Abuse

The elder population experiences abuse and neglect as a vulnerable population. Just as child abuse is underreported, it is estimated that only one out of every 14 cases of elder abuse or neglect are disclosed. Of the reported cases, 10% of the elder adult population (60 years and older) living at home suffer abuse, neglect, or exploitation. The victims are 66% female versus 34% male. For adults with disabilities, 30% who use Personal Assistance Services (PAS) reported one or more types of abuse by their PAS provide (National Council on Aging, 2019).

Similar to the child population, neglect is the most common form of elder abuse. Passive neglect or failure to provide the victim with life's necessities accounts for 58.5% of reported cases. Willful deprivation or deliberately denying life's necessities is another form of neglect. It is estimated that 5.1% of cases are reported for exposing the adult to risks of physical, mental, or emotional harm (National Council on Aging, 2019).

Physical abuse is the second largest reported form of elder abuse. 15.7% of reports cite infliction of physical pain or injury upon an adult. The third likely form of abuse covers 12.3% of reported cases and includes financial exploitation, misuse, or withholding adult's resources to the disadvantage of the victim and/or to the advantage of another person. Verbal assault or threats were identified as emotional abuse in 7.3% of cases. Sexual abuse accounts for 4% of reports and includes inappropriate touching, fondling, or other sexual activity with an adult, when the person is unable or unwilling to consent, or is threatened or physically forced (National Council on Aging, 2019).

Identification & Screening

Screening Questions

- Has anyone at home ever hurt you?
- Has anyone ever touched you without your consent?
- Has anyone taken anything that was yours without asking?
- Has anyone refused to give you your medication, kept you from taking it or given you too much or too little?
- Have you ever signed any documents that you didn't understand, or you didn't want to sign?
- Are you afraid of anyone at home?
- Has anyone taken or broken something you need to be independent, such as your cane, walker or wheelchair?
- Are you alone a lot?
- Has anyone ever failed to help you take care of yourself when you needed help?

Information adapted from Center on Elder Abuse (2019).

Best Practices in Screening

- Screen privately without caregivers/family
- Make eye contact with patient
- Speak slowly and reassuringly
- Become familiar and comfortable with screening questions
- For positive screen, make an intentional hand off to internal/external resources
- Consider CCP211 completion for impaired adult patients

Source: Information adapted from Center on Elder Abuse (2019).

Characteristics of Abuser

The abuser profile is equally distributed on a gender level in reported cases with estimates of 51% are women and 49% are men. Abusers may have a history of substance abuse, aggressive behavior, and undiagnosed or under controlled mental illnesses. Abuser behavior can shift between blaming the victim for the abuse or attitudes of indifference, complaining of a lack of assistance, or painting themselves as the victim in the situation. The abuser usually doesn't allow the victim to speak to or be alone with others and gives conflicting accounts of incidents when questioned. Healthcare providers may also note a significant non-compliance with the prescribed care plan, medication, and follow up visits, as these may be managed by the abuser (Center on Elder Abuse, 2019).

Red Flags

Child Populations

Abuse

- Unexplained or questionable scars, burns, welts, bruises, or fractures
- Unnecessary confinement
- Witnessed beatings
- Sexual abuse
- Emotional abuse
- Withdrawn, angry, or unusual behavior exhibited by the child

Neglect

- Malnourishment, failure to thrive and grow
- Lack of medical care
- Filthy or unsafe environment
- Poor hygiene and personal care
- Absence of parents/appropriate supervision
- Irregular school attendance

Source: Information adapted from National Children's Alliance (2020).

Adult Populations

Abuse

- Witnessed beatings
- Emotional abuse
- Sexual abuse
- Unexplained or questionable scars, burns, welts, bruises, or fractures

- Signs of unnecessary confinement
- Financial exploitation

Neglect

- Hazardous housing
- Failure to administer prescribed medications or seek medical care for the adult
- Any situation where there is failure to provide for the needs of the adult that result in physical harm to that person

Source: Information adapted from National Council on Aging (2019).

Where Do I Report Abuse or Neglect?

The following is an example of the different agencies to report suspected abuse and neglect based on the identified population. The resource below references the agencies for the state of Illinois. It is considered best practice for CMs to collect contact information for similar resources for your practice area and create a single reference for easy access.

DCFS (age birth to about 18 years) | 800-252-2837

Office of Inspector General (disabled, 18-59) | 800-368-1463

Senior Services (if from home or independent living) | 866-800-1409

IDPH (if from nursing home) | 800-252-4343

Self-neglect

- < age 60 | OIG 800-368-1463 (may not take report)
- > age 60 | 866-800-1409

Domestic violence, rape 18-59

- No mandate reporting for this population
- Resources statewide
- www.aardvarc.org/dv/states/ildv.shtml

Source: Information adapted from Illinois Department on Aging (2015).

What to Report?

Sometimes making the actual call can be overwhelming because it may be unclear what detailed information is need for the report. Prior to making the call, gather information you're your impressions of the situation to make a thorough and efficient report. The checklist below can serve as a guide for organizing your report.

- Reason for allegation of abuse/neglect.
    - What is triggering the report?
    - Patient condition, patient report of abuse, report of abuse from a 3rd party?
- Your assessment of risk of harm to adult.
    - Report your observations.
- Mental/physical condition of alleged abuser, if known.
- Location of alleged victim's residence.
- Identity/location of witnesses, if any identified.
- Whether you agree to be contacted for additional information.
    - Reports can be made confidentially in most cases.

Case Study 7.3

Mrs. Johnson is a 75-year-old female, presenting to the emergency department (ED) with complaints of a possible urinary tract infection (UTI). An assessment demonstrates a disheveled presentation, dirty clothes, multiple small wounds and "scratch marks" on her arms, legs and trunk. Her medical records shows that she has had four visits to the ED in the last two weeks for the same complaint.

The ED CM visits with her in the to discuss the previous plans of care. A prescription for antibiotics were given each time and appointments for follow up with primary care physician were scheduled. Mrs. Johnson states she does not know if the prescriptions were filled, "maybe I lost them." When asked if she saw her primary care physician during this time, she states "my daughter-in-law is working, I don't have a ride, and I am watching my grandchildren while she's at work." When she is asked about the scratch marks and wounds on her body, she in-forms the CM that she is "always itchy." A mini mental exam demonstrates that Mrs. Johnson is alert, oriented to person and place (knows she is at the hospital, but cannot name the hospital) and is not oriented to the day, date, or time. Mrs. Johnson is placed in observation status for treatment of UTI and altered mental status.

The CM in the ED makes a report to Adult Protective Services (APS) for possible neglect, based on the multiple ED presentations, not being provided with appropriate follow up such as medication and a physician appointment, the suspicion of insect infestation in the home, and concern over the childcare situation in response to Mrs. Johnson's current altered mental status.

APS receives the report and makes arrangements to gain access to home and investigate. Upon initial investigation, the report is confirmed for neglect and discharge planning for short term nursing home placement for rehabilitation and safety are made. Referrals for community services for alternative childcare arrangements, pest control, and family counseling were made to support the family and prepare for Mrs. Johnson's desire to return to the family home.

References

Bullock, L. F., Sandella, J. A., & McFarlane, J. (1989). Breaking the cycle of abuse: how nurses can intervene. *Journal of Psychosocial Nursing and Mental Health Services, 27* (8), p.11-15.

Center on Elder Abuse. (2019).

Illinois Department of Aging. (2015). Elder Abuse and Neglect Handbook, 2015 edition.

National Children's Alliance. (2020). National Statistics On Child Abuse.

National Council on Aging. (2019). Elder Abuse Facts.

HUMAN TRAFFICKING: CONSIDERATIONS FOR THE PROFESSIONAL CASE MANAGER

Introduction

After drug dealing, human trafficking is tied with the illegal arms trade as the second largest criminal industry in the world, and it is the fastest growing. Every year, human traffickers generate billions of dollars in profits by victimizing millions of people in the United States and around the world. Traffickers are estimated to exploit 40.3 million victims with an estimated 25 million victims in forced labor and 15 million victims in sex trade or forced marriage. Despite growing awareness about this crime, human trafficking continues to go underreported due to its covert nature, misconceptions about its definition, and a lack of awareness about its indicators (National Human Trafficking Resource Center, 2019).

Definitions

Human trafficking is a crime involving the exploitation of someone for the purposes of compelled labor or a commercial sex act through the use of force, fraud, or coercion. Human trafficking affects individuals across the world, including here in the United States, and is commonly regarded as one of the most pressing human rights issues of our time. Human trafficking affects every community in the United States across age, gender, ethnicity, and socioeconomic backgrounds. Human trafficking is a form of modern-day slavery in which traffickers use force, fraud, or coercion to control victims for the purpose of engaging in commercial sex acts or labor services against his/her will (National Human Trafficking Resource Center, 2019).

Sex Trafficking

The recruitment, harboring, transportation, provision, or obtaining of a person for a commercial sex act, in which a commercial sex act is induced by force, fraud, or coercion, or in which the person induced to perform such an act has not attained 18 years of age (United States Code (2000); 22 USC § 7102).

Commercial sex act induced by force, fraud or coercion, or in which the person performing the act is under age 18. Victims can be found working in massage parlors, brothels, strip clubs, or for escort services.

Labor Trafficking

The recruitment, harboring, transportation, provision, or obtaining of a person for labor or services, using force, fraud, or coercion for the purpose of subjection to involuntary servitude, peonage, debt bondage, or slavery (United States Code (2000); 22 USC § 7102).

Victims can be found in domestic situations as nannies, maids, sweatshop factories, janitorial jobs, construction sites, farm work, restaurants, and forced panhandling rings.

Trafficking is a crime that exploits the victim. The physical movement of the victim is not a requisite. Victims are not only women but can be men and children as well.

Pertinent Definitions under United States Code (2000); 22 USC § 7102

Force involves the use of rape, beatings, and confinement to control the victim. Forceful violence is used especially during the early stages of victimization, known as the 'seasoning process,' which is used to break the victims' resistance to make them easier to control.

Fraud usually involves false offers of employment. For example, women and children will reply to advertisements promising jobs as waitresses, maids, and dancers in other countries and are then forced into prostitution once they arrive at their destinations. Fraud may also involve promises of marriage or generally a better life.

Coercion involves threats, debt-bondage, and psychological manipulation. Traffickers often threaten victims with injury, death, or the safety of the victim's family back home. Many trafficking victims are also controlled through 'debt-bondage' in the context of paying off transportation fees into the destination countries. Traffickers commonly take away the victims' travel documents and socially isolate them to make escape more difficult.

Victims often do not realize that it is illegal for traffickers to dictate how they have to pay off their debt. In many cases, the victims are trapped into a cycle of debt because they have to pay for all living expenses in addition to the initial transportation expenses. Fines for not meeting daily quotas of service or "bad" behavior are also used by some trafficking operations to increase debt. Most trafficked victims rarely see the money they are supposedly earning and may not even know the specific amount of their debt. Even if the victim's sense that debt-bondage is unjust, it is difficult for them to find help because of language, social, and physical barriers that keep them from obtaining assistance.

International Impact

Approximately 800,000 to 900,000 victims annually are trafficked across international borders worldwide. Between 18,000 and 20,000 victims are trafficked into U.S. annually. More than half of the victims trafficked into United States are thought to be children and are adults are both women and men (United States Department of State, 2019).

Victims can be trafficked into the U.S. from anywhere in the world. Within the U.S., both citizens and non-citizens can fall prey to traffickers. Trafficking victims sent to the U.S. typically do not speak

English. They often are unable to communicate with service providers, police, or others who might be able to help them.

Victims of trafficking are often kept isolated, and their activities restricted in order to prevent them from seeking help. They are typically watched, escorted, or guarded by the traffickers themselves or associates of the traffickers. Traffickers also may "coach" their victims to answer questions with a cover story about being a wife, student, or tourist. Victims of trafficking often comply with their traffickers and are afraid to seek help because they are in fear for their lives and the lives of their families back in their native countries (United States Department of State, 2019).

Trafficking Victims Protection Act of 2000 (TVPA)

In the U.S., the Trafficking Victims Protection Act of 2000 (TVPA) defines labor trafficking as, "the recruitment, harboring, transportation, provision, or obtaining of a person for labor or services, through the use of force, fraud or coercion for the purpose of subjection to involuntary servitude, peonage, debt bondage or slavery" (United States Code (2000); 22 USC § 7102).

Areas of Focus:
- Prevention
    - Public awareness and education
- Protection
    - Trafficking or "T" visa, certification, benefits, and services to help victims rebuilt their lives
- Prosecution
    - Created federal crime for trafficking, new law enforcement tools and efforts
- Enables trafficking victims to obtain medical care, witness protection, other types of social service assistance
- Enables victims to obtain legal immigration status
- Criminalizes trafficking
- Permits prosecution where victim's service compelled by confiscation of documents
- Increases prison terms for all slavery violations from 10 years to 20 years; adds life imprisonment for death, kidnapping or sexual abuse of victim

The TVPA was just the beginning of federal legislation to address human trafficking. The Preventing Sex Trafficking and Strengthening Families Act of 2014 seeks to reduce the incidence of sex trafficking among youth involved in the foster care system. The William Wilberforce Trafficking Victims Protection Reauthorization Act of 2008, Trafficking Victims Protection Reauthorization Act of 2013, and the Frederick Douglass Trafficking Victims Prevention and Protection Reauthorization Act of 2018 each renew the original TVPA principles, protections, and penalties (U.S. Dept. of State, 2019).

Accessing Services under TVPA

The TVPA provides a means for non-citizen victims in the U.S. to apply for a special visa (T-Visa) and other benefits and services so that they can safely and securely rebuild their lives.

- Temporary status in US
- Recognizes that return to their country of origin may not be in their best interests and gives the opportunity to rebuild without threat of deportation
- After three years, can apply for permanent status

Victims who are U.S. citizens are already eligible to receive many of these benefits. Adult victims of human trafficking (age 18 and over) who are certified by the U.S. Department of Health and Human Services (HHS) can receive federally funded services and benefits to the same extent as refugees. To receive certification, an individual must: be a victim of human trafficking as defined by the TVPA, be willing to assist with the investigation and prosecution of traffickers, and have completed a bona fide application for a T visa or have received Continued Presence status from the U.S. Department of Homeland Security (United States Code (2000); 22 USC § 7102).

Child victims of human trafficking (under age 18) are immediately eligible for benefits. They do not need to apply for a T visa or get Continued Presence status. They are issued "letter of eligibility" from DHHS, no certification process is needed.

Identification & Intervention

- How do we identify potential victims?
- How do victims navigate through this process?
- How do they learn about their rights as victims?
- How do they obtain the necessary documentation and complete the required forms in order to access the services that they need?

This is where the role of the CM becomes critical throughout the duration of a case, whether the victim is male or female, an adult or child, or international or domestic.

- Healthcare providers play an important role in identifying and helping trafficking victims
- While trafficking is a largely hidden social problem, victims are in plain sight if you know what to look for
- There are very few places where someone from outside has opportunity to interact with a victim

A person who is trafficked may look like many of the people you help every day, seeking care from all types of healthcare environments for all different levels of care. Sensitively asking the right questions and looking beneath the surface will help you identify those people who have been forced or coerced into a life of sexual exploitation or forced labor. While the victim may appear to you as a prostitute or a willing participant, look for the following clues:

- Is the person accompanied by another person who seems controlling? This may be the trafficker or someone working for the trafficker.

- Does the person accompanying the person insist on giving information to you?

- Can you see or detect any physical abuse? Does the person have bruises or other signs of battering?

- Does the person exhibit submissive or fearful behavior in the presence of others?

- Does the person have difficulty communicating with you because of language or cultural barriers?

- Does the person have any identification or documentation?

In one study, 87.8% of trafficking survivors reported accessing healthcare services during their trafficking situation. Of these victims, 68.3% were seen at an emergency department (Lederer & Wetzel, 2014).

"During the time I was on the street, I went to hospitals, urgent care clinics, women's health clinics, and private doctors. No one ever asked me anything anytime I ever went to a clinic."

– Lauren, survivor
(Lederer & Wetzel, 2014)

Red Flags from the Relias (2016)

- **Common work and living conditions**
    - Is not free to leave or come and go as he/she wishes
    - Is in the commercial sex industry and has a pimp or manager
    - Is unpaid, paid very little, or paid only through tips
    - Works excessively long and/or unusual hours
    - Is not allowed breaks or suffers under unusual restrictions at work
    - Owes a large debt and is unable to pay it off
    - Was recruited through false promises concerning the nature and conditions of his/her work
    - High security measures exist in the work and/or living locations (e.g. opaque windows, boarded up windows, bars on windows, barbed wire, security cameras, etc.)

- **Poor mental health or abnormal behavior**
    - Is fearful, anxious, depressed, submissive, tense, or nervous/paranoid
    - Exhibits unusually fearful or anxious behavior after bringing up law enforcement
    - Avoids eye contact
- **Poor physical health**
    - Lacks medical care and/or is denied medical services by employer
    - Appears malnourished or shows signs of repeated exposure to harmful chemicals
    - Shows signs of physical and/or sexual abuse, physical restraint, confinement, or torture
- **Lack of control**
    - Has few or no personal possessions
    - Is not in control of his/her own money, no financial records, or bank account
    - Is not in control of his/her own identification documents (ID or passport)
    - Is not allowed or able to speak for themselves (a third party may insist on being present and/or translating)
- **Other**
    - Claims of just visiting and inability to clarify where he/she is staying/address
    - Lack of knowledge of whereabouts and/or of what city he/she is in
    - Loss of sense of time
    - Has numerous inconsistencies in his/her story

As a professional CM, it is important to understand the mindset of trafficking victims.

- They are often confined to room or small space where they eat, work, and sleep.
- They fear and generally don't trust many providers, the government, police, or authority figures.
- Victims may feel that their current situation is their fault, and guilty feelings for their situation.
- Trafficking victims may develop loyalties and positive feelings toward their trafficker as way to cope with their situation – known as the Stockholm or Patty Hearst Syndrome. In these cases, they may even try to protect the trafficker from authorities.
- Traffickers frequently move their victims to escape detection. As a result, trafficking victims may not even know what city or country they're in.
- Victims of trafficking also fear for the safety of their family members who are often threatened by the traffickers.
- They may not speak English or understand U.S. culture (Clawson & Dutch, 2015).

Case Study 7.4

Meera comes to the ER with severe stomach pain. A man identifies himself as Meera's uncle and offers to translate for her. He explains that although she has had "female problems" recently, she has not been to a doctor because she doesn't have insurance. Meera does not make eye contact with ER staff or her uncle. A nurse explains to Meera's uncle that she needs to examine each patient privately, and the uncle says something harshly to Meera in Hindi.

Through the interpreter, Meera informs the nurse she helps clean her uncle's house and provides childcare for other family members. While she loves her family, Meera is stressed because she works 16 hours every day. She is constantly being watched and is not allowed to use the phone or mail letters to home by herself.

Hospital staff diagnoses Meera with a stomach ulcer and writes her a prescription. Obviously troubled, Meera says she's been to another ER before and had the same diagnosis. She stopped taking the medicine because she had trouble saving enough money to pay for the medication, and she is unable to go to a pharmacy without her uncle's assistance.

Adapted from New York City Human Trafficking site (2015).

Special Considerations

There are a number of special considerations you should keep in mind when working with a potential or known trafficking victim.

Before questioning a potential trafficking victim, it is vital to isolate the individual from the person accompanying him or her. However, try to do this without raising suspicions of the individual accompanying the person, who may say they are a spouse, other family member, or employer. This individual may actually be the trafficker. You may want to say that your organization's policy is to talk to people one-on-one.

Case Study 7.5

Heather comes to a clinic for an HIV screening. Although her intake paperwork says she is 20, the nurse observes that developmentally, she seems far younger. Heather tells the nurse she's mature for her age and very experienced. She also has a tattoo on one arm with symbols from a local gang. During the exam, she constantly receives texts and calls to her cell phone. She answers the phone and says 'Baby, don't worry, I'll be done soon.' She tells the nurse her boyfriend, Sam, is so in love with her that he can't be away from her for even one minute.

The screening results indicate that although Heather is HIV negative, she has multiple other sexually transmitted infections (STIs). The nurse asks Heather whether she uses protection during sex, but she shrugs and says, 'Sometimes they don't want to.' When the nurse asks who 'they' are, Heather says that sometimes she has sex with other men but does not elaborate. She says it won't be forever, just until she and her boyfriend can save up some cash for a place of their own."

Adapted from New York City Human Trafficking site (2015).

It is also important to enlist a trusted translator or interpreter who also understands the person's cultural needs. Don't rely on the individual accompanying the person to translate, since this individual could be the trafficker and will likely sanitize the person's responses. If the person is a child, it is important to call in a specialist skilled in interviewing children who are trafficking or abuse victims.

Trafficking victims are often in intense danger (or their families could be in danger) if they try to leave their situations. As a result, strict confidentiality is paramount. Therefore, talk to the person in a safe, confidential, and trusting environment and limit the number of staff members who come in contact with the trafficking victim.

The person may initially deny being a trafficking victim out of fear, and it is best not to ask direct questions. Instead, indirectly, and sensitively probe the person with sample questions such as:

- Can you leave your work or job situation if you want?
- Has anyone threatened your family?
- Do you have to ask permission to eat, sleep or go to the bathroom?

- When you are not working, can you come and go as your please?
- What are your working or living conditions like?
- Is there a lock on your door or windows so you cannot get out?
- Have you been threatened with harm if you try to quit?
- Where do you eat and sleep?

Adapted from National Human Trafficking Resource Center (2019).

Gaining trust with the trafficking victim will be an important first step in providing much-needed assistance to this individual. This graphic gives sample messages you may want to convey to trafficking victims to help gain this trust and demonstrate that you care for their well-being and safety.

Victims of human trafficking are vulnerable human beings who have been subjected to severe physical and emotional coercion. These trafficking victims are usually in desperate need of assistance. They need to know that once they come into contact with social service providers, they should feel protected and safe.

There are benefits and services available to trafficking victims including legal, healthcare, counseling, housing, food, medical, cash and employment assistance. A toll-free number has also been created for reporters to call if you think you have encountered a victim of trafficking. By calling the Trafficking Information and Referral Hotline, you can help identified victims of trafficking get this assistance.

References

American Bar Association. (2016). Victim Assistance Fact Sheet.

Clawson, H. & Dutch, R. (2015). Case management and the victim of human trafficking: a critical service for client success. Department of Health & Human Services.

Futures Without Violence. (2015). Case Management Approaches to Support Trafficked Victims. OVW Training.

National Human Trafficking Resource Center. (2019). Human Trafficking & Healthcare Settings.

National Human Trafficking Resource Center. (2019). Recognizing and Responding to Human Trafficking in Healthcare. National Human Trafficking Resource Center.

New York City. (2015). Human Trafficking Example Cases.

Relias Media. (2018). Human Trafficking is a Problem for Case Managers and All HCWs.

State of Illinois. (2018). What Is Human Trafficking?

U.S. Department of State. (2019). International and Domestic Law; Office to Monitor and Combat Trafficking in Persons. https://www.state.gov/international-and-domestic-law

United States Code. (2000); House of Representatives. 22 USC § 7102(9) Trafficking Victims Protection.

Resources

National Human Trafficking Resource Center www.TraffickingResourceCenter.org

United States Law on Human Trafficking https://uscode.house.gov/view.xhtml?path=/prelim@title22/chapter78&edition=prelim

THE IMPACT OF THE IMPACT ACT OF 2014

The IMPACT Act was signed into law on October 7, 2014 but was finalized on September 28, 2019 and implemented on November 29, 2019. IMPACT stands for Improving Medicare Post-Acute Care Transformation Act of 2014.

Four Goals

- GOAL: to standardize the information collected between four post-acute care providers (PACs)
    - Inpatient Rehabilitation Facility (IRF)
    - Skilled Nursing Facility (SNF)
    - Long Term Acute Care Hospital (LTACH)
    - Home Health Care Agencies (HHC)
- GOAL: data collected is to be interoperable so as to allow exchange of data and information between the PACs
- GOAL: to improve quality of care across the provider settings and reduce readmissions
- GOAL: to improve hospital and discharge planning

Background

CMS's Conditions of Participation (CoP) for Discharge Planning requires the hospital provide discharge planning services to help manage transition from hospital to home or other healthcare setting. Discharge planning includes determining the appropriate post hospital destination for patients by identifying what the patient requires for a smooth, safe transition and beginning process of meeting the patients identified post discharge needs. This includes an assessment of any social determinants of health (SDoH) disparities.

Patient Choice

The Discharge Planning CoP specifies the process for discharge planning assessment and addresses collaboration with a patient to meet their post discharge needs. Commonly referred to as "patient choice," this is the directive to ensure patient collaboration and involvement in the discharge planning process. The CoP specifies that, as part of the discharge planning process, the CM must inform the patient or the patient's family of "their freedom to choose among participating Medicare providers of post-hospital care services and must, when possible, respect patient and family preferences" when they are stated, without limitations or bias of providers. (CMS, 2013).

A process to facilitate this freedom of choice is outlined in the CoP:

> the hospital must include in the discharge plan a list of post-acute service providers of all types that are available to the patient, that are participating in the Medicare program, and that serve the geographic area in which the patient resides, or, specifically in the case of a SNF, in the geographic area requested by the patient (CMS, 2013).

This "choice list" is given to all patients for whom post-acute services are indicated and have been determined to be appropriate by the discharge planning evaluation and collaboration with the multidisciplinary care team. Distribution of the "choice list" must be documented in the medical record along with the patient's preference of post-acute providers.

Significance

Consider the IMPACT Act was designed and signed in 2014, 2013 Discharge Data of Medicare Beneficiaries was used as background information (Centers for Medicare and Medicaid, 2019).

- 8 million discharges to Post Acute Care (PAC)
    - 84.9% of discharges to SNF
    - 76.2% of discharges to LTAC
    - 68.7% of discharges to IRF
    - 64.6% of discharges to HHC

Patients with inpatient stays who discharge to post-acute care can experience longer stays and more costly episodes of care than patients who were discharged directly to home with outpatient follow-up—7 days and 3.6 days respectively. The average cost of care is twice as much when a patient is discharged to post-acute services ($16,900) versus when the patient is discharged home with outpatient follow-up ($8,300) (Centers for Medicare and Medicaid, 2019).

At a time when the U.S. is in the middle of a population "boom" becoming eligible for Medicare services, the need for connecting patients with high quality, low-cost services in the post-acute space is vital to the survival of Medicare. According to the report "The Value of Home Care" by the Home Care Association of America and the Coalition on Aging:

- By 2020, 56 million Americans will be aged 65 and older
- By 2050, 84 million Americans will be aged 65 and older
- Americans over 85 years of age is on pace to triple by 2040
- Nearly 70% of Americans who reach 65 will be unable to care for themselves at some point without assistance (HCAOA, 2016).

IMPACT Act Key Points

1. The biggest change is the requirement that hospitals apply the discharge planning process to *all* patients, including inpatients, outpatients under observation status, outpatients undergoing sedated procedures or surgery, and emergency department patients identified as needing a discharge plan.

   • GOAL: ensuring that more patients who might experience complications and costly readmissions are identified.

2. Requires that a copy of the discharge instructions and the discharge summary be sent to the practitioner responsible for the patient's follow-up care within 48 hours of discharge; test results must be communicated within 24 hours of their availability.

   • GOAL: smoothing transitions and ensuring that patients receive timely follow-up care.

3. Includes a new requirement that hospitals establish a post-discharge follow-up process to check on patients who return home. The rule does not prescribe a follow-up strategy or specify the timing of these activities, leaving hospitals flexibility to design their own programs.

   • GOAL: better care coordination, reduction of readmissions.

4. In addition to giving patients lists of post-acute care providers, hospitals must help patients and their caregivers select providers by using and sharing data on quality and resource use measures as required by the IMPACT Act.

   • GOAL: utilizing high quality providers to expedite recovery and movement along the continuum of care to lower levels of care more effectively.

It is this requirement we will focus on because of the challenges it poses for the professional case manager. Challenges such as understanding of "who does what" in the post-acute realm

   • Hampers the ability of the CM professional to communicate clearly with patient/family
   • Referral to inappropriate level of care
   • Lack of providing a continuum of care/support that progresses
       - Acute Hospital to SNF to Home Health to Home Care
       - Acute Hospital to LTACH to Hospice with Home Care
   • How to get quality data without adding more steps, paper to DCP process
   • How to educate patient/families on needs and what they can realistically provide

Patients traditionally select post-acute providers based on:
   • Geographic proximity to home
   • Word of mouth recommendations from friends/family
   • Perceived comfort with facility/staff
   • Most are unaware of publicly available quality data for these providers of care

- IMPACT ACT requires that, in addition to giving patients lists of post-acute care providers, hospitals must help patients and their caregivers select providers by using and sharing data on quality and resource use measures.

The Discharge Plan under the IMPACT Act must now address the following:

- The physician or practitioner responsible for the patient must be involved in the process of establishing the patient's goal of treatment

- The plan must be patient-centered and address the patient's preferred treatment preferences.

- The plan must consider the support person or caregiver's capacity to perform the required care and the patient's ability to perform self-care as well.

- The plan must consider what care is available in the community including addressing social determinants of health disparities.

- The discharge planning team (including the patient/caregiver) must include access CMS publicly reported quality metrics for review when selecting post-acute care providers (available at Medicare.gov).

Best Practices

The question is how exactly does the CM include these goals in the discharge planning process? It requires engaging the patent/caregiver in the process and appropriate selection of the suitable level of care with the correct level of care provider based on the quality data that is available. The quality data is readily available on Medicare.gov at Nursing Home Compare, Home Health Compare, and other search engines on the Medicare website. How do we make it available, understandable, and actionable for our patients/caregiver to be able to use it effectively?

Accountable Care Organizations (ACO)

Accountable Care Organizations have been leaders in utilizing high quality, low-cost providers. ACOs are provider led organizations that have a strong base in primary care and are accountable for quality and the cost of care across the continuum. Because of this accountability, they create network of pre-approved post-acute care providers for their members based on quality metrics.

Partner Provider Networks

Provider networks can be created in a less formal environment than an ACO. This is an informal group of providers gathered by a central entity (usually a hospital) are invited by the hospital to participate as part of the team providing continuing care services with a sharp eye towards quality. Inclusion in these networks can be based on home grown criteria, but always include the CMS quality data as the foundation.

Software/Database

Less formally, facilities can use software or databases to help access the CMS quality search engines at Medicare.gov to collaborate with the patient and the family members in selection of post-acute providers. Technological solutions eliminate the need for continuously printing potential provider selections on a case-by-case basis from Medicare.gov. Additionally, software or database options can enable the patient or CM to email other decision-makers directly from the portal with the information to be considered in choosing a post-acute provider.

Impact of IMPACT

The IMPACT act uses data available to facilitate better outcomes at lower cost to all patients. The CMs now take a more active role in the discharge planning process with a focus on quality in the best interests of our patients and take the pre-2014 "patient choice" requirement to a new level of "informed patient choice" through education and advocacy.

Key Takeaways

- The patient and caregiver/support person must BOTH be involved in the development of the discharge plan.

- The patient and caregiver/support person must be informed of the final plan and agreement must be documented.

- The discharge plan MUST address the patient's goals and treatment preferences

- Such as patient is having major foot surgery and wants to recover at home while physician prefers a rehab center (SNF)

- The hospital must assist patient and their family in selecting a post-acute service provider, including using/sharing data about home health agencies, SNF, IRF, LTACH, and Hospice providers on quality and resource use measures. This data must be relevant to the patient's goals and treatment preference

- The discharge plan must be included in the patient's medical records.

References

Burke, R., Whitfield, E., Hittle, D., Min, S., & Levy, C. (2015). Hospital readmission from post acute care facilities: Risk factor, timing and outcomes. *JAMDA*, December, 2015.

Centers for Medicare and Medicaid. (2019). Hospital Conditions of Participation for discharge planning: 42 CFR §482.43,

Centers for Medicare and Medicaid. (2019). State Operations Manual, Appendix A – Survey Protocol, Regulations and Interpretive Guidance for Hospitals, Rev. 151, November 20, 2015, p. 412.

Centers for Medicare and Medicaid. (2019). "CMS-Approved Accrediting Organizations, Contacts for Prospective Clients," September 2, 2015.

Centers for Medicare and Medicaid. (2019). Revision to State Operations Manual, Hospital Appendix A – Interpretive Guidelines for 42 CFR 482.43, Discharge Planning, p. 413.

Centers for Medicare and Medicaid. (2019). Improving Medicare Post-Acute Care Transformation Act of 2014, Public Law 113-185, October 6, 2014, 128 STAT 1960.

Cesta, T. (2016). Case management's role in the new proposed bundled payment program. *Hospital Case Management, 24*(4), 51-54.

Home Care Association of America. (2016). The Value of Home Care.

Mennella, H. A. (2016). Discharge Planning: United States Centers for Medicare and Medicaid Services (CMS). *CINAHL Nursing Guide.*

New discharge planning rules focus on preferences, transitions. (2016). *Hospital Case Management, 24*(2), 17-20.

Pellett, C. (2016). Discharge planning: Best practice in transitions of care. *British Journal Of Community Nursing, 21*(11), 542-548.

Schub, E. B. (2016). Patient Discharge and Discharge Planning: Government Regulations. *CINAHL Nursing Guide.*

Weissenstein, E. (1997). New post-acute rule takes effect, but HCFA regs absent. *Modern Healthcare, 27*(45), 70.

Wrobleski, D. S., Joswiak, M. E., Dunn, D. F., Maxson, P. M., & Holland, D. E. (2014). Discharge Planning Rounds to the Bedside: A Patient- and Family- Centered Approach. *MEDSURG Nursing, 23*(2), 111-116.

Resources

Conditions of Participation for Discharge Planning https://www.govinfo.gov/content/pkg/CFR-2007-title42-vol4/pdf/CFR-2007-title42-vol4-sec482-43.pdf

Impact Act https://www.govinfo.gov/app/details/CREC-2014-09-18/CREC-2014-09-18-pt2-PgS5862-5

BUNDLED PAYMENTS FOR CARE IMPROVEMENT (BPCI)

High Level Overview

Bundled Payments for Care Improvement (BPCI) was an initiative created by the Center for Medicare and Medicaid Innovation (CMMI) to test the efficacy of several different episode-based payment models with three goals in mind:

- producing higher quality care
- providing more coordinated health care
- lowering the cost of care to Medicare

The original BPCI program was launched in 2013 and it concluded in 2018. The BPCI Advanced (BPCI-A) Model is a new iteration of the program and a continuation of efforts to implement episode-based payment models, also referred to as bundled payments.

Bundled Payments and BPCI

As a review, in traditional fee-for-service (FFS) payment models, providers are paid for each individual service they furnish to patients for a single illness or course of treatment. Bundled payments provide a single, comprehensive payment that covers all services provided during a patient's episode of care (services provided to a beneficiary with a medical condition within a specific time frame and across the continuum of care).

Each of the four BPCI models had significant differences in which portions of the continuum of care were included (hospital, post-acute care, primary care), as well as in how payments were made, and discounts calculated. Variances include:

- Who is eligible to participate in the model?
- Clinical conditions included for consideration
- Included services (various combinations of inpatient, post-acute, and readmissions)
- Expected discount calculations
- How the provider will be paid
- Which quality measures will be evaluated for the model?

BPCI provider participants choose from one of four models to participate in, and three of the four models gave providers the ability to further specify which of 48 different clinical episodes/diagnosis group they would participate within (Center for Medicare and Medicaid, 2019).

Examples of these Inpatient Clinical Episodes/Diagnosis Groups include: (not all inclusive)

- Stroke
- Sepsis
- Cardiac Arrythmia
- Renal Failure
- Cellulitis
- Acute Myocardial Infarction (AMI)
- Urinary Tract Infection (UTI)
- Gastrointestinal Hemorrhage
- Gastrointestinal obstruction
- Congestive Heart Failure
- Simple Pneumonia & Respiratory Infections
- Chronic Obstructive Pulmonary Disease (COPD), Bronchitis, Asthma
- Disorders of the Liver, (excluding malignancy, cirrhosis, and alcoholic hepatitis)
- Major joint replacement of upper or lower extremity
- Coronary Artery Bypass Graft (CABG)

BPCI Advanced (BPCI-A)

The Bundled Payments for Care Improvement Advanced (BPCI-A) Model is the new iteration of BPCI. BPCI-A aims to continue to build on the successes of BPCI, while making appropriate changes and improvements to correct gaps identified in the original BPCI program.

Some important updates include:

- A wider view of the episode of care – the duration of all clinical episodes now includes the anchor (initial) stay + 90 days, while the original BPCI program allowed participants to choose from 30- 60- or 90-day bundles.
- Fewer exclusions are allowed – all Part A services resulting from the Anchor (initial) Stay/ Procedure are included, as well as post-acute services, including home and hospice care. Participants must expand their cost and quality efforts to include services previously excluded from the bundle.
- BPCI Advanced will qualify as an Advanced Alternative Payment Model (Advanced APM) through the Medicare Access and CHIP Reauthorization Act (MACRA) – this could incentivize physician group practices and hospital-employed physicians to participate in order to avoid payment adjustments under the Merit-based Incentive Payment System (MIPS) (Center for Medicare and Medicaid, 2019).

This newest update to the concept of alternative payment models (APM) and value-based care demonstrates that they are here to stay. CMs should know which APM their facility is participating in, the specifics about which patient populations are included, and required notification of participation to the patient (Center for Medicare and Medicaid, 2019).

Notification to the Beneficiary/Patient

The beneficiary must be notified the facility is participating in BPCI-A. The CMS Beneficiary Notification Letter is a requirement of the BPCI Advanced Participation Agreement. As part of a Beneficiary Notification Plan, the facility should provide the Beneficiary Notification Letter to each patient identified by diagnosis as a BPCI Advanced Beneficiary prior to his or her discharge from an inpatient stay or completion of an outpatient procedure (Center for Medicare and Medicaid, 2019).

The goal of the letter is to "communicate the existence and purpose of the BPCI Advanced Model, the BPCI Advanced Beneficiary's right of access to medically necessary covered services, and the beneficiary's right to choose any provider or supplier for covered services" (Center for Medicare and Medicaid, 2019). The letter may not be modified from the template provided by CMS but may be translated into other languages as long as the content stays the same.

References

Center for Medicare and Medicaid (2019). Bundled Payments for Care Improvement Advanced Frequently Asked Questions.

Resources

Bundled Payments for Care Improvement Advanced Frequently Asked Questions. https://innovation.cms.gov/media/document/bpci-advanced-generalfaq-my5

Bundled Payments for Care Improvement Advanced Notification Letter and Instructions https://blogs.cooperhealth.org/ctd/files/2018/10/BPCI-Advanced-Beneficiary-Notification-Letter-template_v2.pdf

THE BASICS OF PATIENT TEACHING

Jeff Crofoot MSN RN CMCN ACM-RN

Patient education is an essential function in the role of a CM. Identified knowledge deficits must be addressed to promote optimal patient outcomes and decreased readmissions. This may range from simply directing a patient to take their medication to making major lifestyle changes leading to an improved level of health and quality of life (Muma, 2012). Education is the first step towards the patient's ability to self-manage their health condition.

Resource material can be found on the Agency for Healthcare Research and Quality's (AHRQ) website. Effective methods are important as studies have shown that as much as 80% of the information given to patients during an office visit is forgotten at once or is incorrectly understood (AHRQ, 2020). Low health literacy can affect the patient's compliance with medical care ultimately leading to poor patient health outcomes (AHRQ, 2017).

The CM may be the best resource for patient education. Physicians are rarely taught communication skills during their training and may overestimate their own skills. Communication tends to be more focused on empathy and using plain language rather than actual patient teaching. One study showed that medical residents reported using the teach-back method 60% of the time, while it was observed to occur only 2.5% of the time (Feinberg, 2019). Communication is a core competency for doctors, both MDs and Doctors of Osteopathy (DOs), yet neither program includes health literacy.

Patient teaching should occur when there is a change in their health needs. This can include a new diagnosis, new medications, recommended lifestyle changes, use of a new device, or when there are new treatment options. Patient teaching should occur not only when there are changes but also when the patient is having recurrent problems with an established diagnosis. For example, repeated readmissions for the same medical diagnosis may indicate a lack of understanding.

Consider the condition of the patient. Assess for language barriers. Use a medical interpreter when available and appropriate. If hearing impairment is observed, speak in a lower tone (not lower volume), avoid extraneous noises, minimize distractions, and enunciate clearly. Speak slowly as processing speed for new information may decline with age. You may need to decrease the amount of new information being presented. In all cases, involve the caregiver whenever possible and speak using age-appropriate terms.

When teaching, do not appear rushed and allow time for the interaction. Remain approachable and encourage the patient to ask questions. Speak to the patient at eye level. Sit down next to the patient and don't hover over them. Remove physical barriers, such as your computer or a desk that are between you and the patient. Maintain a positive attitude and be aware of the tone of your voice. Do not appear frustrated if the patient fails to understand. These steps will foster a more relaxed environment conducive to learning. Initiate the teaching prior to the time of discharge. Once patients are aware that they are being discharge, their focus is often not on the material but rather leaving the hospital.

Teach-Back

Teach-back is an evidence-based method which ensures the information has been explained clearly so the patient and family not only understand, but are able explain the new knowledge in their own terms as opposed to simply repeating what they were told (AHRQ, Teach-Back: Intervention., 2017). The patient is literally teaching back to the CM what they have learned. This validates the teaching intervention was successful, and the patient clearly understands the new information.

Simply asking a patient if they understand will often yield a positive response even when there is not clear understanding. The patient may be too embarrassed to say do not understand or may believe they do but have misinterpreted the information. There are several advantages to using the teach-back method. It helps the patient better recall the information discussed. The patient will feel more relaxed and less anxious about the new material. Patient satisfaction will be higher and fosters a more trusting relationship between the patient and nurse case manager (AHRQ, 2020).

The method should not be viewed as a quiz or test for the patient but rather a way to validate the effectiveness of your teaching interventions and alert you that your communication may not have been clear. The teach-back method has been shown in studies to have better outcomes than group classes in terms of self-management skills (Namratha, 2011). Class instruction tends to be unidirectional. Group settings may discourage questions, especially those with low health literacy. There can be a disconnect linking the new information and patient activation of that information. The teach-back method slows the flow of information and makes the process more interactive and does not require a great deal of resources. It can be performed without a need for additional staff. For staff well trained in the method, in can add only a few minutes to the interaction, yet yields great results in terms of patient education. The only other additional cost is for the printed materials provided to the patient.

There are a few key points to remember when using the teach-back method.

- **Start with the most important message or point you are trying to convey.** This may include the need for a certain medication, dietary restriction, or steps for medication administration.

- **Limit the conversation to two to four keys points,** and lead with the most important point. Too much information all at once can be overwhelming or confusing to the patient and lessen overall recall. It may be necessary to rephrase or restate points to ensure understanding.

- **Use plain language and avoid medical terms.** Use terms such as "reduces swelling" instead of "anti-inflammatory" and "high blood sugar" instead of "hyperglycemic."

- **Use demonstration to assess for comprehension.** For tasks such as blood sugar monitoring or inhaler use, have the patient not only demonstrate the task but be able to provide the case manager with instructions in their own words.

- **Return demonstration should also be used.** Examples include proper use of inhaler or incentive spirometer or performing blood sugar testing. Start with a phrase such as "show me how you will use your inhaler at home" and then allow the patient to demonstrate step by step. Prior to beginning, inform the patient that afterwards you will be asking them to demonstrate or explain the information provided.

- **Evaluate for patient understanding.** Rephrase until the patient can explain the information in their own terms, essentially "teaching back" the information to the case manager.

If upon evaluation, the patient is unable to teach-back or demonstrate the skills after your teaching intervention, you will need to alter your approach. Do not allow the patient to feel as though they have failed. Use phrases such as "I must not have done a good job explaining this. Let me try it this way." This does not assign blame to the patient for failing to understand, which can lead to greater anxiety on the patient's part. If a verbal only approach did not work, use drawings or demonstrate the skill needed.

EDUCATE Model

The EDUCATE model is an acronym for a 7-point model (Marcus, 2014). The steps do not necessarily occur sequentially but may be approached simultaneously during the flow of the conversation. The model incorporates the use of teach-back strategies.

"**E**" is for enhancing comprehension and retention. The patient should have a list of questions to ask for better understanding. Repeat the important points and ask the patient to repeat back in their own words. Provide information in several different ways such as verbally and with written handouts in simple language, avoiding complex medical terms.

"**D**" is for delivering patient-centered education. The use of empathetic skills when the patient's view of the situation differs from the facts of the situation. The CM pursues a greater understanding of the patient's viewpoint. Seek information about the patient's life experience as it relates to the health issue being discussed. Ask about the patient's concerns and work to dispel them.

"**U**" is for understanding the learner. Assess what the patient knows already. Start at basic level as the patient may not even be aware of their misunderstandings and knowledge deficits. You can approach this with simple questions to gauge their understanding of disease process, medications and treatments. Assess for any health literacy barriers, such as language, that may impede the teaching process. Involve the patient's family or care givers when possible and with the patient's consent.

"**C**" is for communicating clearly and effectively. Lead with the most important information first, but with no more than three key points. Present the information in logical way that builds on mastered knowledge. Keep language simple and avoid complex medical terms. Use concrete examples relevant to the patient whenever possible. Encourage and allow the patient to ask questions. The types of questions can be used as a gauge of understanding. Use a qualified interpreter when language barriers are identified.

"**A**" is for addressing health literacy and cultural competencies. While asking the patient if they need assistance understanding information about their health and treatment, do not stop if the patient answers "yes." Ask the patient to explain in their own words. Written material should be supplemental and a reinforcement to verbal instruction and not a replacement for the direct verbal interaction.

"**T & E**" are for teaching and education goals. Preparation is important and clear goals serve as a measurement of success. A planned teaching approach and written teaching materials can enhance the success. Use teachable moments. These occur when the patient is not feeling rushed or anxious. Teaching should occur throughout the stay and not at only at the moment of discharge.

NEAT Model

NEAT is an acronym for Nurse Education and Transition. Like the EDUCATE model, it also incorporates the teach-back method. The goal is not to teach everything but instead focuses on what is termed as the "survival skills" needed at the time of transition home from the hospital (Krall, 2016). The steps include assessing the patient's needs, prioritizing the information vital for the transition home, selecting appropriate materials, providing materials and teaching to the patient, assessing the knowledge gains, providing a list of "survival skills" once home, and setting up further teaching interventions. The method, like teach-back, focuses on a few main points. In the case of diabetes, the main focus points would be nutrition, medications, insulin injections, blood sugar monitoring and awareness of the effects of hypoglycemia.

Summary

Learning can be defined as a change in long term memory (Namratha, 2011). When new information is learned, it is incorporated with existing knowledge and changes the way the person thinks about the concept. Heath literacy can affect this as those with low health literacy have less of a starting point and require greater learning to reach the overall objective. A common characteristic of the teaching methods presented is using simple language and avoiding complex medical terms. Involve the patient's family or caregiver whenever possible.

The CM must be able to evaluate the success of the teaching interventions to ensure patient understanding. A patient's understanding of their disease process, treatment, proper use of medical interventions and medications is fundamental to their overall health. The ability to understand and self-manage their conditions is vital to positive health outcomes.

References

AHRQ. (2017, April). *Agency for Healthcare Research and Quality.* Retrieved from teach-back interactive module slides.

AHRQ. (2017, December). *Teach-Back: Intervention.*

AHRQ. (2020, September). *Health Literacy Universal Precautions Toolkit.*

AHRQ. (2020, September). *The Share Approach.*

Center for Medicare and Medicaid. (2018). *Are you Hospital Inpatient or Outpatient?*

Case Management Society of America. (2010). *Standards of Practice for Case Management.* Little Rock,Arkansas: Case Management Society of America.

Feinberg, I. E. (2019). Perception versus reality: The use of teach back by medical residents. *Health Literacy Research and Practice*, 118-126.

Fink-Samnick, E. (2019). *The Essential Guide to Interprofessional Ethics in Healthcare Case Management.* Brentwood, TN: HCPro.

Krall, J. D. (2016). The nurse education and transition (NEAT) model: Educating the hospitalized patient with diabetes. *Clinical Diabetes and Endocrinology.*

Marcus, C. (2014). Strategies for improving the quality of verbal patient and family education: a review of the literature and creation of the EDUCATE model. *Health Psychology and Behavioral Medicine*, 482-495.

Medicare Advantage 2020 CMS Inpatient Only List. (2020).

Medicare and Medicaid Programs; Revisions to Requirements for Discharge Planning for Hospitals, Critical Access Hospitals, and Home Health Agencies, and Hospital and Critical Access Hospital Changes to Promote Innovation, Flexibility, and Improvement (2019, September 20).

Medicare Benefit Policy. (2005, December 16).

Namratha, K. E. (2011). Literacy and retention of information after a multimedia diabetes education program and teach-back. *Journal of Health Communication*, 16:89-102.

Patient Experience Institute. (2021, February 28). *About.*

The Beryl Institute. (2021, February 28). *The Beryl Institute.*

Resources

Agency for Healthcare Research and Quality. Teach-back interactive module slides: https://www.ahrq.gov/patient-safety/reports/engage/interventions/teachback-mod.html

Agency for Healthcare Research and Quality Health Literacy Universal Precautions Toolkit. https://www.ahrq.gov/health-literacy/improve/precautions/tool5.html

Agency for Healthcare Research and Quality. The Share Approach. https://www.ahrq.gov/health-literacy/professional-training/shared-decision/index.html#:~:text=AHRQ's%20SHARE%20Approach%20is%20a,about%20the%20program%20is%20available

PATIENT EDUCATION: ONE CASE MANAGER'S STORY

Mariana Turgeon MSN RN BSCS CCM

Patient education and case management education go hand in hand. It is my experience that CMs are expected to have a solution to most, if not ALL of the issues on the unit that pertains to discharging patients. Many of these barriers can be resolved through patient education.

Discharge barrier – An RN was discharging her patient and going over discharge instructions. The patient let the RN know after discharge instructions were given that they had NO ride home or they had called a friend or family member to pick them up, but they hadn't heard back. At the same time, the beds are filling up and the nurse manager keeps walking around to see if the patient has discharged yet.

Education provided to the patient included that many insurance plans have transportation benefits. Anyone can look at the back of the patient's insurance card and find out right away if they have that benefit. I have sat with several patients and walked them through the process. In addition, we make sure they have a follow up appointment and guide them in setting up transportation arrangements for that first follow-up appointment.

For example, at my current organization, we have access to a company called Roundtrip. We can schedule an Uber or Lyft to take the ambulant patient home. This company allows us to get the ambulatory patient home safely without having to wait for the insurance transportation window of two to four hours or the use of medical transportation vans or services.

Because of this transportation barrier for some patients, we have modified our initial assessment questionnaire to ask whether they have transportation from the hospital. If there is a transportation issue, most of the MDs know to create a case management referral so we are aware ahead of time and can work on the issue before discharge.

Teaching plays a MAJOR part in dealing with respiratory patients, especially during flu season. Respiratory patients may be prescribed discharge medications like albuterol, DuoNeb and Pulmicort (medications used in nebulizers). Upon assessment, it is found that either they did not have a nebulizer at home or were asked if this medication can be used in their "family member's" nebulizer because the child did not have their own nebulizer. RED flag!

At the time, we had an Asthma Educator nurse practitioner (NP) that would see the patients before discharge and make an appointment to see them in the home. She was noticing the patients she saw in the home many times did not have their own nebulizers. They were using other family members' nebulizers. The team got together and decided that first, we needed to identify at admission if the patients needed a nebulizer. Secondly, we needed to make sure they knew how to maintain the nebulizer at home. In addition, we needed to know if the patient could learn to use inhalers with spacers thus not needing the nebulizer.

I also added a question to my initial CM assessment. "Do you have a nebulizer at home, if so, how old is it or where did it come from?" This is a basic question, but we received many different answers.

- I can borrow one from my grandmother.
- I think we had one, we would have to look for it (the patient was 5 years old).
- We got one from the ER, but we have not used it because we had to send it back and I can't afford to pay for it if it gets broken.

Medication Teaching

The physicians were adamant they wanted the refill medication at bedside BEFORE discharge and wanted to be assured the patients would also have their medications to take home. In filling these medications at bedside, it decreased discharge problems twofold. It flagged prescriptions that were not on the patient's insurance formulary. If not, the pharmacist and I would work with the prescribing MD to obtain authorization or ask the MD to prescribe a similar medication that would be covered.

For medications that are unfamiliar to the CM, take the initiative to research articles about the patient's diagnosis, commonly used medications, and provide your patient with information written primarily for lay person use instead of printing from a medication resource that does not present information in plain language, written at a 5th grade reading level. Remember to consider primary language as well and use resources that offer multiple language translations.

Durable Medical Equipment

To be able to give good patient education on asthma, I started researching articles about asthma and education, and I found a research article that stated that parents were good about administering the asthma medications but tended to forget about the maintenance and upkeep of the machine. The article stated there was a strong possibility that they could inadvertently be reinfecting their children. The potential reinfection was due to small tubing diameter and even running it through water or a cleaning solution did not guarantee the tubing was clean.

I reached out to the DME respiratory therapist, and she stated the nebulizer tubing can be replaced several times a year and all the patients had to do is call the DME provider (usually the sticker on the side of the nebulizer) to ask for a whole new setup. This important piece of information has been folded into the patient education for our asthma patients and has made a positive impact on the patients/caregivers who directly receive the information and their communities because they have passed that information on to others.

Follow-up Appointments

Another research article I found stated families were more likely to attend hospital follow up appointments if the appointment was already made versus if they had to make the appointment themselves. From my perspective, the families were so thrilled that their child was well and being discharged, that many times they forgot to schedule a hospital follow-up with the PCP, pulmonologist, or both. Other studies show that patients do not make their follow up appointments due to lack of engagement, unfamiliarity with the assigned provider, or feeling that they "just saw a bunch of doctors, why do I need to see another one?" (Morley & Walker, 2019).

Case Study 7.6: The Impact of Patient Education

Once during an assessment, I was asking the grandfather who took care of his 10-year-old cystic fibrosis grandson if his grandson had a nebulizer, how old it was, and how often he used it. I stated that I learned parents were great about giving the medication, but sometimes forgot to clean the machine and mask. The grandfather looked at me with a "deer in the head light look." He then turned to his daughter and asked if this "cleaning and maintenance" pertained to CPAPs too. The daughter looked at her father with the weirdest look and asked "Dad, why are you asking?" The grandfather said proudly, "Your mother used to take care of those things." His wife of 50 years had passed away about five years earlier from cancer. At that time, he took on a major role of caring for his grandson.

His daughter stated they did maintain her son's nebulizer, replacing the tubing and mask after every acute illness. She also said she would look at her father's continuous positive airway pressure (CPAP) machine. She asked if we could possibly help with replacing accessories and I said absolutely. Of course, I would work with the grandfather's pulmonologist or PCP to get him what he needed.

On the day of discharge, the daughter brought in her father's CPAP. She would not even handle it without gloves on. She put it in a clear, plastic bag and we could not believe what we saw. The whole inside length of the tubing had a black and gray haze. The daughter had taken the filters out of the CPAP the night before and they were a "charcoal" color (they were supposed to be white). She felt ashamed that her dad had been breathing that in all those years, EVERY NIGHT, because he followed his MD's directions to use the CPAP every night.

I worked with the grandfather, and we were able to get an appointment with his PCP in two days. I was able to order a brand-new CPAP (much smaller than his original one). In addition, we were able to set him up with a new sleep study because since his wife had passed, he had not had an appointment.

Who knew a CM with a labor and delivery background would be able to provide important asthma education to families about the use of their asthma medication, the maintenance of their asthma machine, and ensuring they had appropriate follow up appointments prior to discharge? Unknowingly – we found our asthma education affects others unexpectedly.

To summarize, ANY LITTLE teaching will reach families that need it. At times we feel unheard but those times where just one patient benefits from our teaching makes it all worth it!

PROFESSIONAL ORGANIZATIONS: AN IMPORTANT ELEMENT OF PERSONAL AND PROFESSIONAL DEVELOPMENT

Eric Bergman RN CCM

Healthcare is complex. After all, that is why CMs are so important. However, what if you are the CM? How are you supposed to learn what you need to know to do your job?

Join a professional organization!

Professional organizations are focused on protecting, enhancing, and nurturing specific professions. The complexity of health and healthcare has created a need for specialization, and with that specialization has come the growth of specialized professional organizations. Case management has its own group of professional organizations supporting our specialty.

Professional organizations create conditions and an environment that enhances practice and practitioners through collective work and support. A professional organization allows individuals engaged in similar work at different settings, to gather together for collaboration, mutual support and education. They set standards for practice that define and protect the practice and profession. Standards are most powerful when supported and agreed on by most practitioners and when they guide the practice to protect and benefit the public. By publishing and popularizing standards of practice, professional organizations increase public trust, understanding, and respect for a profession and thereby increase the effectiveness and influence of the professional practitioners.

A good professional organization will gather the leading thinkers, practitioners, and influencers to participate in forums, meetings, and committees, to lead and support the profession. These groups draw on their collective experience and expertise to resolve problems, provide education, influence public policy, refine standards, and mentor new practitioners. The organization then promulgates the results of this collective work through seminars, conferences, white papers, press releases, newsletters, journals, social media and virtual networks.

Standards and Codes of Conduct

Standards of practice or codes of conduct are used to shape and influence training for a profession, as well as to provide a framework for practitioners to evaluate and structure their daily work. "The standards of practice are clearly framed, authoritative statements that distinguish unique responsibilities for which its practitioners are held accountable" (Fink-Samnick, 2019). These standards can also be used to create, and refine job descriptions, support legal practice guidelines for licensure and set the standards for a scope of practice. The standards and codes also provide reassurance to the public the practitioner will adhere to these standards and codes and can therefore be trusted to provide valuable and safe services.

Standards of Practice and Codes of Conduct are living documents which require regular evaluation and updating to remain viable and relevant as new discoveries and advances in our understanding of the professional work we do change the daily practice and expectations. A strong professional organization will have members and leaders who are highly skilled and experienced and who wish to invest in the support of their profession. The professional organization provides an avenue for these thought leaders to gather and collectively review, enhance and refine the standards and codes.

Examples of codes and standards

- Case Management Society of America (CMSA) Standards of Practice
- Commission for Case Management Credentialing (CCMC) Code of Professional Conduct for Case Managers
- The American Case Management Association (ACMA) Transition of Care Standards

Protecting the Profession

The leaders of a professional organization work to protect the profession through the creation and maintenance of standards and codes, but also through the collective work of their members. The organization will dedicate staff and volunteer time to monitor, research and suggest changes to public policy affecting the profession and its clientele. The professional organization will frequently have influence with accrediting or licensing boards by providing model language or promoting leaders to serve on the public committees creating the rules and regulations. In other cases, members are organized to research and publish articles in the organization's journals and newsletters to inform both practitioners and the public about the important work undertaken by the practitioners of the profession. These articles serve not only as educational tools, but also as examples and advertisements of the important work done by the profession.

Sometimes an organization can be effective in influencing public opinion and perception of the profession with media campaigns. For example, by creating and marketing public service announcements (PSAs), such as the Case Management Society of America's video "Ask for a Case Manager"), which are accessible on their YouTube channel and website (CMSA.org). Books that are published by practitioners about their work or blog posts and magazine articles are promoted and distributed by professional organizations to help promote and build the public image of practitioners. Sometimes the organization will publish books of their own to help promote the profession.

Professional organizations also monitor and advocate for title protections for their practitioners. By promoting licensure and certification, professional organizations can limit the practice of the profession to licensed or certified practitioners. These limitations provide a pathway to discipline practitioners who fail to adhere to the standards and laws governing the licensees or certificate holders, and thus instill confidence in the public that they will be protected when engaging the services of a licensed or certified practitioner.

Networking

One of the most valuable benefits of a professional organization is the power of networking. The collaboration and mutual focus of members of the organization can build relationships that enhance and strengthen the work of individuals by helping them to meet, collaborate, and learn. It is powerful to attend conferences and meetings with others who are engaged and interested in the same subjects, activities, and work as you are. Conferences provide opportunities for informal and spontaneous discussion. Lasting friendships grow out of these interactions and collaborative work occurs that provides people with energy, new ideas, and excitement to advance projects, grow personally, and achieve common goals.

A strong professional organization creates opportunities for networking by fostering projects that span the whole of an industry or bring together practitioners who are seeking to achieve common goals from across the country or region. By working together, these groups can achieve far more than if they were attempting the same projects, or experiments in their individual work settings. The power of collaboration often results in outcomes that are far greater than the individual contributions, commonly referred as the power of synergy.

A good professional organization will have a journal and newsletter that provide opportunities for members to publish their work. A high-quality journal will include "peer review" which ensures the studies and projects published are well constructed, meaningful, and reproducible, thus ensuring the quality and value of the work. Members can learn from the research presented and use it to enhance their personal practice or they can gain valuable publicity and help others to improve by publishing their own work.

One of the most valuable aspects of the networking opportunities provided by professional organizations is personal connection. "Social connection improves physical health and psychological well-being" (Seppälä, 2012). "Social connection can lower anxiety and depression, help us regulate our emotions, lead to higher self-esteem and empathy, and actually improve our immune systems. By neglecting our need to connect, we put our health at risk" (Canadian Mental Health Association, 2019). From personal connections we can grow as individuals as well as professionally. Building a strong network within a professional organization can lead to significant career advancement. "Over 80% of job seekers say that their network has helped them find work" (Doyle, 2020). Your network can provide you with advice about improving your resume and point you to employers that are great to work for. They can even help you discern new directions or specializations suited to your interests and skills.

Many professional organizations provide opportunities for mentoring. For new practitioners this is an invaluable resource for career advice and personal growth. For the seasoned professional serving as a mentor, there are many rewards including the satisfaction of helping a new practitioner grow and improve their skills and value to the profession. One of the most powerful tools for strengthening education and understanding is to teach others. As we evaluate and teach, we examine our own knowledge and reflect on our experience. The act of organizing our knowledge and experience into a cohesive and concise package that can be shared with others deepens our own understanding and can frequently lead to improvements in our own practice.

Advocating for Public Policy Improvements

There is great power in numbers. Professional organizations help practitioners congregate and build coalitions either within a single area of practice or by partnering with other organizations to work for a common issue. For example, if I want to advocate for a change in the legal rules about the practice of nursing in my state, I can write a letter to the nursing board or my representatives in the state legislature and ask them to consider my idea. If I am well organized, I will gather a dozen or so of my friends to help. But if I can persuade my professional organization that my idea has merit and get the professional organization to advocate with me, then I can begin to draw on the influence of the whole membership of that professional organization. I can tell legislators and board members that my comments are endorsed and supported by my colleagues in the professional organization. But let's not stop there. If I can further influence my professional organization to partner with other professional organizations whose member may be similarly affected by my recommended change, then I can draw on the power of all those members and build a coalition of many thousands of individuals who can then wield significant influence.

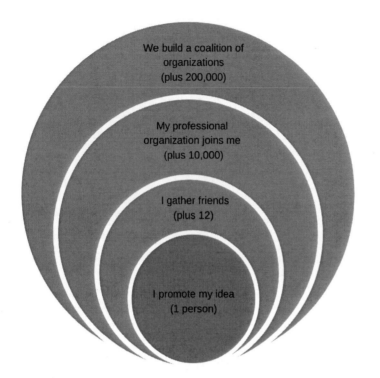

Chart 7.2 The Power of Collaboration

Data and layout of this figure by author.

Another aspect of advocacy that professional organization engage in is providing expert advice and opinion to law makers, media organizations, and the public in general. Through the organization's publications, direct outreach on issues, or by maintaining speakers' bureaus, a professional organization helps to shape public opinion or leaders' understanding of the profession, and important rules, events, or activities related to the profession. The organization brings together industry experts to develop strategy and discuss solutions. The results of these activities are then promulgated by the organization and its leaders to the public, shaping public opinion, rules and regulations, and the practice of the profession. The experts within the professional organization gain recognition, credibility, and influence through their association with a well-organized and respected professional organization.

The focus of an organization's advocacy takes many different forms depending on the needs of the profession or its clients.

Choosing Your Organization(s)

The practice of case management and the organizations that support the work of CMs is enormously varied. To begin with, CMs come from and practice in every area within the healthcare continuum of care. They also are drawn from a wide range of professions, including nursing, social work, physical, occupational, speech, respiratory therapy, pharmacology, and medicine. Healthcare CMs are licensed professionals in one of the fields of medical care, and may be members of a professional organization supporting that practice, such as the American Nurses Association (ANA), or the National Association of Social Workers (NASW). In addition, many practitioners come from specialties within their practice which have their own professional organizations, such as the Association of Rehabilitation Nurses (ARN), the Oncology Nurses Society (ONS), or the American Association of Critical-Care Nurses (AACN). But you have chosen a new area of specialization, case management, and now it is time to decide where you will find the professional support for your new professional home.

As you embark on your search you will discover that there are a large number of professional organizations within case management. Below you will find a table of the various organizations and the URLs for their websites. It is helpful to understand that some of the organizations are membership based professional organizations that provide their own case management certification or credentials, while others partner with standalone certification organizations.

The three largest organizations are (in alphabetical order): ACMA, CCMC, and CMSA. ACMA is a professional organization with membership that also has its own certification subsidiary, which administers and manages the ACMA associated certifications. CCMC is a standalone certification organization without members, but which participates in some of the traditional activities of professional organizations, such as provided educational resources and an annual conference. CMSA is a professional organization that has a membership base who are certified and credentialed by other organizations.

There are at least 12 different certificates aimed at case management professionals, and while not all of them have an associated professional organization, each of the certificates is aimed at practitioners focused on different aspects of the health care continuum. Your choice of professional organization to join could in part be guided by your choice of which certificate you wish to pursue, or which you have already earned. The following table is not a complete listing of every professional organization which supports case management, but it does include most of the largest and well-known.

Professional Organizations for Case Managers[1]

Organization / Focus audience / Associated certifications	PO[2] or CB[3]	# of certificants as of 2020[4,5]
American Board of Managed Care Nursing　www.abmcn.org Focus audience: Health care professionals working in managed care settings[6] Associated certifications: - Certification in Managed Care Nursing - Certified Managed Care Professional	CB	2,400+ combined
American Case Management Association[7]　www.acmaweb.org Focus audience: Case managers in settings that deliver health care including transitions of care[8] Associated certifications: - Accredited Case Management Certification (ACM™) - Case Management Administrator Certification (CMAC)	Both	7,000 ACM 140 CMAC
American Nurses Credentialing Center[9]　www.nursingworld.org Focus audience: RNs who practice case management[10] Associated certifications: - Nursing Case Management Board Certification (CMGT-BC™)	CB	2,066 as of June 2020
Association of Rehabilitation Nurses　rehabnurse.org Focus audience: Nurses working the field of rehabilitation[11] Associated certifications: - Certified Rehabilitation Registered Nurse	Both	~13,000
Case Management Society of America[12]　cmsa.org Focus audience: Licensed health care professionals working as case managers Associated certifications: - None, but collaborates with CCMC and offers continuing education pre-approved by CCMC	PO	n/a

Organization / Focus audience / Associated certifications	PO[2] or CB[3]	# of certificants as of 2020[4,5]
Commission for Care Manager Certification ccmcertification.org Focus audience: RNs, SWs and other allied health professionals[13] Associated certifications: - CCM® - CDMS®	CB	45,000 active 65,000 CCM 2,200+ CDMS
National Academy of Certified Care Managers www.naccm.net Focus audience: Health and human service professionals working in primarily home and community-based care management programs serving adults.[14] Associated certifications: - Care Manager Certified (CMC)	CB	3,214 total 1,348 active
National Association of Social Workers[15] www.socialworkers.org Focus audience: Both bachelors and masters prepared social workers Associated certifications: - Certified Social Work Case Manager (C-SWCM) - Certified Advanced Social Work Case Manager (C-ASWCM)	Both	Data unavailable
Patient Advocate Certification Board www.pacboard.org Focus audience: All individuals in the field of patient advocacy[16] Associated certifications: - Board Certified Patient Advocate	CB	686 as of July 2020
Patient Experience Institute and **The Beryl Institute** pxinstitute.org www.theberylinstitute.org Focus audience: Healthcare patient experience professionals[17] Associated certifications: - Certified Patient Experience Professional (CPXP)	Both	1,200+

Table 7.2 Professional Organizations for Case Managers

[1]The information in Table 7.2 was compiled from a variety of sources, including the organizations' websites, the 2021 Special Report: Stepping Up to Certification by Anne Llewellyn, and The Essential Guide to Interprofessional Ethics in Healthcare Case Management by Ellen Fink-Samnick.

[2]Professional Organization

[3]Certification Board

[4](Llewellyn, 2021 Special Report: Stepping Up to Certification, 2021)

[5]For a detailed and broad explanation for the importance of certification and accreditation as well as thorough discussion of the many organizations providing oversight and certification for healthcare case management, please see Chapter 2 of Ellen Fink-Samnick's The Essential Guide to interprofessional Ethics in Healthcare Case Management. See also Anne Llewellyn's 2021 Special Report: Stepping Up to Certification for detailed information about many of the certificates listed below, including thorough explanations of the history, purpose and scope of each certificate.

[6](American Board of Managed Care Nursing, 2021)

[7]ACMA is the second largest professional organization focused on the practice of case management.

[8](Llewellyn, 2021 Special Report: Stepping Up to Certification, 2021)

[9]ANCC is the certification arm of the American Nurses Association (ANA). Together with ANA, and the ANA Foundation if forms ANA Enterprise. The organization is the largest and most active professional organization for nurses in the united states.

[10](ANA Enterprise, 2021)

[11](Association of Rehabilitation Nurses, 2021)

[12]CMSA is the oldest and largest professional organization focused on the practice of case management.

[13](Llewellyn, 2021 Special Report: Stepping Up to Certification, 2021)

[14](Llewellyn, 2021 Special Report: Stepping Up to Certification, 2021)

[15](Fink-Samnick, 2019)

[16](Patient Advocate Certification Board, 2021)

[17](Patient Experience Institute, 2021)

Conclusion

Whether you are embarking on your career or have years of experience as one of those "helping professionals," as case management thought leader Anne Llewellyn refers to us, you will need support and resources to grow your professional practice and network. "Our healthcare system is complex, fragmented, costly, and at times unsafe. Having professionals in place who can assist consumers navigate through the healthcare maze is important" (Llewellyn, 2021 Special Report: Stepping Up to Certification, 2021). Finding the right professional organization will enrich your professional life, improve your practice, and likely change the trajectory of your career for the better.

Professional organizations offer the support and education necessary to excel in today's complex and ever-changing health care world. In order to perform well as a CM, you must have extensive education and a wide variety of resources because your clients' issues are complex. You will more fully meet their needs, if you are able to draw on the enormous resources you will gain through membership in a good professional organization.

References

American Board of Managed Care Nursing. (2021, February 28). Home.

American Case Management Association. (2019). *Transitions of Care Standards*.

ANA Enterprise. (2021, February 28). About Us.

ANA Enterprise. (2021, February 28). *Nursing Case Management Certification* (CMGT-BC).

Association of Rehabilitation Nurses. (2021, February 28). Home.

Canadian Mental Health Association. (2019, October 17). *The Importance of Human Connection*.

Case Management Society of America. (2010). *Standards of Practice for Case Management*. Little Rock, Arkansas: Case Management Society of America.

Cherry, K. (2021, January 7). *Psychosocial Development Guide*. Retrieved from VeryWellMind.com: https://www.verywellmind.com/generativity-versus-stagnation-2795734

Commission for Case Management Credentialing. (2015, January). Code of Professional Conduct for Case Managers. Mount Laurel, New Jersey, United States of America.

Doyle, A. (2020, August 5). *The Importance of Career Networking*.

Fink-Samnick, E. (2019). *The Essential Guide to Interprofessional Ethics in Healthcare Case Management*. Brentwood, TN: HCPro.

Llewellyn, A. (2018). *The 2018 Special Report: Stepping Up to Certification: A Case Manager's Guide to Certification*. Fort Lauderdale, FL: Blue Bayou Press, LLC.

Llewellyn, A. (2021). *2021 Special Report: Stepping Up to Certification*. Fort Lauderdale, FL: National Academy of Certified Care Managers. (2021, February 28). Home Page.

Patient Advocate Certification Board. (2021, February 28). Home.

Seppälä, E. (2012, August 26). *Connect to Thrive*. Psychology Today.

The Beryl Institute. (2021, February 28). *The Beryl Institute*.

Thompson, B. D. (2017, October 19). *The Upsides and Downsides of Telecommuting*.

PROFESSIONALISM IN CASE MANAGEMENT

Anne Llewellyn MS BHSA RN-BC CCM CRRN

Case management is a practice that is made up of professionals from various disciplines and different experiences. One thing we all have in common is the desire to make the healthcare system patient and family-centered, safe, efficient, and cost effective. We do this is various ways, through patient engagement, patient and family education, timely and safe transitions of care, care coordination, utilization management, and improving communication throughout the broad healthcare system and various stakeholders.

Professional CMs are leaders and use the experiences they bring from their respective fields to do their work. This chapter covers the various requirements professional CMs must have to be successful in their chosen area of practice.

Licensure

We come to the practice of case management from specific disciplines and educational preparation. Many of us are required to hold a license to show that we have met the requirements for our specific discipline. Knowing the scope of practice for your professional discipline is the first step to ensuring the people who care for patients across the broad continuum of care are trained and able to do work they are asked to do. These rules are different for each discipline as well as the states where they live and work, so it is incumbent upon each professional to know the rules of their specific discipline and State Regulatory Agency that oversees their area of practice.

Case in Point: I live in Fort Lauderdale, Florida and hold a Florida license as a Registered Nurse (RN). This license gives me the privilege to work in any area of the healthcare industry as a Registered Nurse. If I take a job as a nurse CM working for a company that requires me to work across state lines, I need to know the rules of the specific state where I am asked to work and to comply with those rules. I may need a license in each state that I work in depending on the requirements. In addition, I may be able to do certain procedures in one state, but not in another. As a professional nurse, I am responsible for knowing and following the rules of the state where I am working.

In 1999, the National Council of State Boards of Nursing (NCSBN) became the first organization to develop and implement two interstate compacts to reduce regulatory barriers to cross-border nursing practice for licensed practical/vocational nurses, registered nurses, and advanced practice registered nurses. The compacts were intended to move from the traditional single-state license to a state-of-residence license allowing the licensee to practice in other participating states. At the writing of this chapter, there are currently 34 states which have enacted NLC legislation, meaning they recognize the multi-state license or have such legislation pending. Other disciplines are working toward their own compact. As a professional, it is important to follow this legislation.

Liability Insurance: Having your own professional liability insurance is important for all professionals to maintain. A CM does not necessarily need to make an error or cause harm to be named in a lawsuit. Most professionals think because they work for an organization they are covered. The organization where you work can refuse to represent you if they perceive you did not follow a policy or procedure and there is a lawsuit.

A client or a client's family member who perceives wrongdoing can file a lawsuit, which can cause a CM financial harm as they work to defend themselves or get dismissed from the lawsuit. A CM can be cautious and meticulous in their practice and documentation, yet still find themselves named in a lawsuit. Having your own coverage is important. A malpractice policy will provide you with representation at depositions as well if you are called before your State Board or the Certifying Body if your certification is in jeopardy. HPSO, which is part of the Nurse Service Organization, offers liability insurance for professionals involved in case management.

Certification: As CMs advance in their careers, many look to achieve national certification. Choosing the right certification to match your goals and expectations is important. Today there are several national certifications that CMs can choose. As you contemplate certification, ask yourself, will being certified:

- Help you professionally?
- Give you job security?
- Help you do your job better?
- Give you an opportunity for professional growth?
- Add credibility to your work?
- Pay you more?

If you can answer yes to these, then certification may be a good choice for you, and you should explore the various certification to see which one benefits you the best. If you can't answer yes to them, you might want to do some reflection as to what you are looking for certification.

Once you decide you want to step up to certification, you will need to choose the national certification that is best for you, apply, and once accepted plan out time to study. Taking a certification is challenging, as most are national in scope and test that you know the fundamentals of the practice across all aspects of case management. If you have been in a specialty area, you might not have the broad knowledge you need for your certification of choice, but you can study to gain that knowledge. Remember, certification tests the basic knowledge of the practice. As an experienced professional, a review of the principles, standards and tools of the practice should help you tackle the certification exam of your choosing.

To assist those looking at national certification, I invite you to check out a Special Report I wrote to help professionals explore the various national case management certifications. In 2021, I expanded the report to include Patient Advocacy and Patient Experience certification as they are emerging professions that many people are choosing. To get your copy, visit my website, Nurse Advocate at https://nursesadvocates.com. Click on the Resource Tab and you will see the 2021 Special Report: Stepping Up to Certification. You can download for free after you enter your name and email address. (Link in Resources List at the end of this section.)

Continuous Learning

As healthcare professionals, CMs need to employ continuous learning into their daily lives. As you know, the only constant in healthcare is that it will change. Staying up to date with those changes is a challenge that each of us has to work out in our own way.

Here are some of the common ways for professionals stay up to date:

Formal Learning: Many professionals choose to go back to school to advance their careers. The basic level for most professions is a bachelor's degree. Many look to attaining a Master's Degree in the field or a complementary field of practice. Today, Doctor of Nursing Practice (DNP) or PhDs are being sought by many as they advance in their careers. Explore these options to see which one is best for you.

Informal Learning: Informal learning is practiced by professionals in many ways. Many read professional journals, e-letters or participate in list-serves or other online portals and groups specific to the area of practice they are in.

Community Organizations/Service Organizations: Others join committees where they work on in their community to use their expertise to educate and empower others in specific areas of practice. Many belong to service organizations as a way to give back to the community.

Professional Organizations are also important ways professional CMs can grow as leaders and experts in an area of practice. There are a number of case management organizations that professionals can join. Doing so is an important part of your professional development.

Continuing Education: As a licensed Registered Nurse and triple Board-Certified CM, I am required to continuously learn. This is part of the requirements to maintain my license and national certification, so I am always on the lookout for ways to do this. I accomplish this by reading articles, attending local, state, and national conferences, and by educating others. Authoring articles, chapters, blogs, and other mediums that pertain to the work I do is another way to earn credit. Case In Point: I can use this chapter as one of my professional education activities when I renew my license or national certification.

Always check the educational requirements for your professional license or national certifications so that you are aware of any specific requirements you need to have, as well as the number of credits you need when renewal time comes along.

There are several ways to collect these credits. As Director of Client Services for Athena Forum, I have been impressed with the rigor and depth of their programs. As a member of the Case Management Society of America, I have access to their educational library and can take an unlimited number of programs to gain continuing education credits for the time I spend reading and learning new material. There are several companies that also offer continuing education programs, so take time to find the one's that fit your area of practice.

One tip is to make sure the number of credits is clearly stated and if they are pre-approved for the certification bodies you need to renew. Most conference committees and educational companies do this as part of the fee you will pay to access the programs, but some don't— leaving you to pay for the course and the continuing education credits.

Pre-Planning: Being certified is an expense that needs to be planned out over time, so it is not overwhelming. Most certification give you an option to retake the test or renew by continuing education credits. The time frame can range from one to three years. Professional license renewals are usually biannually. The fee is set by the state and can be renewed by continuing education. Renewal fees are viewed by professionals as the cost of doing business for most of us. Pre-planning can help you spread the costs over a period of time.

Organization: Being organized is important as you will collect continuing education credits from several sources. Most certifying bodies have a portal or a way for you to track your credits, but if you hold multiple licenses or certification, it can get confusing as these systems don't talk to each other. Having a folder where you can collect all of your continuing education credits in one place, by year, will make it easier when you renew your professional licenses and national certifications. If you are audited, you will need to produce the actual certificate, so hold on to them for at least six years.

Retirement: As you look at retirement, many organizations allow you to hold your certification credentials for a nominal fee—so check out those options. Most require you to show that you are fully retired and are no longer working to fit the criteria. Many professionals may want to work after they formally retire in a part time or per-diem position. If it is not a financial burden, maintain your professional license and national certification until you are sure you no longer need them.

Resources

Nursing Licensure Compact: https://nursinglicensemap.com/resources/nursing-licensure-compact/#:~:text=The%20Nursing%20Licensure%20Compact%20(NLC,of%20NLC%20states%2C%20see%20below.

CMSA Standards of Practice www.cmsa.org/sop

Professional Liability Insurance Information https://www.hpso.com

Anne Llewlellyn's Report: Stepping Up to Certification http://nursesadvocates.com/resources

Epilogue

My intention was to create an "everyday resource guide"—your "go-to" for the "whys and hows" of what we do on a daily basis. It is my fond hope this book serves as an excellent foundation for all the different responsibilities the acute care case manager has every day. The world of acute care case management is many faceted and can be overwhelming at times.

"Start by doing what is necessary; then do the possible;
and suddenly you are doing the impossible."

– St. Francis of Assisi

The quote above from St. Francis of Assisi is an apt comparison to the role of the professional case manager in the acute care setting. Learning to prioritize and organize is paramount to success in acute care case management.

I have tried to include not only the perspective of the acute care case manager, but also those who support us in our quest to provide support and services across the healthcare continuum for our patients. Know that you are not alone but are part of a very large community with one goal and one purpose: to provide excellent patient-centered care.

Keep in mind is that healthcare is ever-changing. Changing Medicare rules, changes from the managed care organizations, other external forces, and internal changes add up. It is imperative you, as the professional case manager, never stop learning. One of the more exciting changes to consider is that case management, long the "best kept secret in healthcare," is finally being nudged into its rightful role on the healthcare team, and what we as a profession have long known is becoming clear to others...the case manager role is VITAL to the success of the patient and the healthcare continuum.

My departing thoughts and tips:

1. Change is constant. Change can be difficult, but it is not going away. Learn to get comfortable with the concept of change. Keep up-to-date with changes and they will not take you by surprise.

2. Continuing education should not just be something you do because you "have to." Be inquisitive. Learn something new.

3. Every piece of the case management process is crucial. Do not trade off one for another. Everything will suffer in the end.

4. Case management data is important. Your documentation is important. Don't skimp on your documentation but don't feel you need to write *War and Peace* about every interaction. Learn to write your notes concisely.

5. Become well-versed in your electronic health care record and documentation system. It will save you time and frustration in the long run.

6. Be a preceptor or mentor. Pass along your knowledge. Share the resources you discover.

7. And lastly, because this concept should be the first and last thought we have in what we do every day…the patient/family is the reason we exist. Giving excellent patient-centered care is what we do, every day, every patient, every encounter.

Please email me with ideas, suggestions for updates, and topics for future editions. I look forward to hearing from you.

Colleen M. Morley
DNP RN CCM CMAC CMCN ACM-RN
cmmorley@altrahealthcareconsulting.com

Case manager…because super amazing, life-changing,
multi-tasking miracle worker isn't an official job title.

(Unknown)

Index

Contributor's Index

My undying thanks to the team that contributed to this book by sharing their expertise and experiences.

Kathy Samas Allen RN CCRN CCM

Kathy is a graduate of Gateway Technical College, Kenosha, WI, University of Wisconsin at Kenosha and University of Texas at Arlington. She has worked in Racine, WI; Milwaukee, WI; Fort Worth, TX; Nashville, TN; and Clearwater, FL.

Her specialties include: Critical Care, ER, PACU, Open Heart, Nursing Administration, Home Care Coordination, Quality Improvement, Infection Control, Corporate Leadership, EMR and Case Management. She is presently living in the Tampa Bay, FL area, working with Post-Acute Case Coordination Management. Her interests include exploring the beautiful Florida beaches, shelling and music.

Anne Albitre LMSW CCM

Anne Albitre LMSW CCM is a Social Work Case Manager providing transitions of care and complex case management in North Texas. She has case management experience in managed care, non-profit, primary care, and behavioral health.

Her expertise includes care transitions and assisting patients navigating the healthcare system to knock down one barrier at a time. She has a strong interest in facilitating new programs and innovative patient care.

She has experience driving innovative projects, including spearheading a contract between a Medical/Behavioral Health Clinic and Hospital in Reno, Nevada to provide safe hospital discharges and reduce readmission rates.

Anne is a member of Case Management Society of America Dallas Fort Worth. She received her MSW from University of Nevada, Reno, and BA in Psychology and BS in Child Learning and Development from University of Texas, Dallas.

Cassandra Battle BSN RN CCM

Cassandra Battle BSN RN CCM current position is Nurse Disease Case Management with Anthem Insurance Company. Prior to this role, she has held positions as center manager with Centra PACE (Program of All-Inclusive Care for the Elderly).

She oversees multiple disciplines across the continuum of the healthcare spectrum to render care to the geriatric patient. She developed her love for the health profession over 21 years ago when she became a certified nursing assistant and wanted to know more. This led to her going back to school to become a licensed practical nurse (LPN) where she served in community base settings, completing home visits and maintaining multiple supervisor positions.

In 2010 she went back to nursing school for an associate's degree as a registered nurse. She worked acute care/medical/surgical units at the bedside. In 2016, she completed her Bachelor of Science in Nursing degree. In 2020, she became a certified case manager.

Cassandra continues to mentor to nursing student candidates. She is also a motivational speaker, and coach to multiple nursing students at the local community college. She recently enrolled into Master of Nursing program. Her husband of eight years and extended family has been and continue to be a strong support to her throughout her nursing and case management education and career.

Eric Bergman BA RN CCM

Eric Bergman RN BA CCM is an International Nurse Case Manager for AXA Partners, one of the world's leading travel assistance companies. He is based in AXA's Chicago office where he has worked as a chronic disease case manager for U.S. expatriates a travel assistance case manager overseeing the evaluation and coordination of care all over the world for patients struck by sudden illness while abroad, and as a repatriation escort, using his expertise in both nursing and international travel to safely move ill patients home.

After receiving a BA in history from Boston University, Eric worked as a flight attendant and union leader for American Airlines for 27 years. In the early 2000's, as the airline industry experienced its worst downturn in several decades, Eric made a mid-life career change and became an RN. His initial nursing experience was inpatient hospice and oncology, where he worked at a community hospital in suburban Chicago for five years.

Eric has served on the Case Management Society of America, Chicago Chapter (CMSA Chicago) Board of Directors since 2014 and currently serves as Past President of CMSA Chicago. He served two terms (June 2018 - June 2020) as Presidents' Counsel Representative for the national organization which includes a seat on the National CMSA Board of directors. Eric also has significant past experience serving on boards of several non-profit organizations, and as a leader of various local and national organizations including as CEO of a not-for-profit educational foundation, treasurer of several service organizations, and manager of local and national political campaigns.

Dr Meghan Bisping DPT PT

Meghan Bisping, PT, DPT is the Director of Rehabilitation Services for West Suburban Medical Center in Oak Park, Illinois for Pipeline Health. The Rehabilitation Department provides therapy services on the acute medical/surgical floors, the 50-bed licensed subacute rehabilitation housed within the walls of the hospital, and at the River Forest Medical Campus Rehabilitation and Sports Medicine Center. Previous roles include: • Senior Physical Therapist for West Suburban Medical Center • Interim Senior Physical Therapists for Holy Family Medical Center • Physical Therapist II for Loyola University Medical Center. Meghan has 10 years of experience as a physical therapist.

Her clinical experience has been focused on the following patient populations: oncology/hematology, lymphedema, ventilator-dependent, minimally responsive/coma stimulation, geriatrics, and COVID-19. Meghan's focus has been the creation and implementation of the Early Mobility Program at WSMC on the medical/surgical floors, including ambulation of ventilated patients in the ICU.

Jeff Crofoot MSN RN ACM-RN CMCN

Jeff earned his nursing diploma from Evangelical School of Nursing in 1987, his BSN from Jacksonville University in 2011, and his MSN from Grand Canyon University in 2015. He has been involved in case management since 1995, working in home care, acute care, and for private insurance companies. Clinical experience includes Medical-Surgical, ICU, home care, infusion and subacute care. He has presented on case management topics on the local and national level.

Janet Coulter MSN MS RN CCM

Janet S. Coulter, MSN, MS ,RN, is a certified case manager. She has been a staff nurse, charge nurse, nurse educator, nurse administrator, case manager, case management team leader, and Director of Case Management for a managed care organization. Janet holds a Master of Science in Nursing from West Virginia University, Morgantown, WV; and a Master of Science in Adult Education from Marshall University, Huntington, WV.

She has been very active in the Southern Ohio Valley Chapter of CMSA, serving as a founding member, board member, Vice President, President-Elect, Secretary, and Chairperson of numerous committees. In addition, Janet has served three terms as President, chairperson of the Fall 2015 Conference, and is currently serving a fourth term as President.

Janet has been active in CMSA at the national level as well. She has presented concurrent sessions and posters at several CMSA Annual Conferences. She was the 2012-2013 CMSA Chapter Presidents' Council Representative on the CMSA Board of Directors, has served as a CMSA Board member, and has participated in or chaired several CMSA Committees. She is currently Secretary of the CMSA Board of Directors, a member of the CMSA Executive Committee, and on the Editorial Board of CMSA TODAY. Janet was the recipient of the CMSA 2015 National Award of Service Excellence, the 2012 Southern Ohio Valley CMSA Case Management Leadership award, and was nominated for the 2012 Case-In-Point 4th Annual Platinum Award, Disability Manager category. She has published many articles in CMSA TODAY and Professional Case Management and was a reviewer for the Core Curriculum for Case Management Third Edition.

Erin Cunningham BSN RN CCM

Erin Cunningham BSN RN CCM is the Regional Director of Case Management for Critical Illness Recovery Division with Select Medical. Prior to this role, she has held positions in acute care as case manager, facilitating utilization review, interdisciplinary team care coordination, and bedside nurse. Erin held a unit manager position for a 63 skilled bed long term care facility facilitating MDS, managed wound care, and developed an ongoing plan of care for residents.

Erin has over 20 years of nursing experience. Her clinical specialties include Med/Surg, Geriatrics and wound care. She received her ADN at Miami University in Oxford, Ohio and BSN at Miami University in Oxford, Ohio.

She is passionate about education and sharing knowledge of resources to ensure the healthcare community is connected and up to date with all available services to ensure a sustainable service for the population we serve. Erin believes it is an honor and privilege to be a part of a patient's healthcare experience.

Erin served as a Board Member for Fort Wayne chapter in 2008 and is currently a Director on their BOD. Throughout the years of membership with Fort Wayne Chapter, Erin offered her support and talents to the Education Committee.

Teri Dreher RN iRNPA CCM BCPA

Teri Dreher is a nationally recognized leader in the emerging field of professional patient advocacy. In 2011, she left a long career in critical care nursing to form NorthShore Patient Advocates, now one of the country's largest professional advocacy companies. Teri is also the founder of Seniors Alone Guardianship and Advocacy Services, a non-profit organization that serves senior orphans and disabled adults. To date she has founded three national advocacy programs, including the International Conference on Patient Advocacy.

Ellen Fink-Samnick MSW ACSW LCSW CCM CCTP CMHIMP CRP DBH(c)

Ellen Fink-Samnick is an award-winning healthcare industry subject matter expert and Principal for EFS Supervision Strategies, LLC. Known as the "Ethical Compass" of professional case management, Ellen is the author of books, articles, and knowledge products. Her academic appointments include the University of Buffalo School of Social Work and George Mason University's Department of Social Work. Ellen is a permanent panelist on Monitor Monday, contributor to Talk Ten Tuesday, and editorial advisory board member for Professional Case Management, Case Management Monthly, and RAC Monitor. Ellen also serves as Lead for Rise Association's Social Determinants of Health Community.

Deanna Cooper Gillingham RN CCM

Deanna Cooper Gillingham RN, CCM is a leader in case management with over a quarter century of experience in healthcare as a registered nurse and case manager. She uses her years of training and expertise, as well as her direct and to the point writing style to make complex information easy for the reader to grasp. Her popular book CCM Certification Made Easy: Your Guide to Passing the Certified Case Manager Exam, now in its 3rd edition, has helped thousands of case management professionals obtain their certification.

As co-founder and CEO of Case Management Institute, LLC, Deanna is developing the case management workforce through her books, courses, and events. Her Foundations of Case Management Course provides nurses transitioning into case management with a firm foundation of the practice. Her Facebook group, Case Managers Community, provides a place for networking and support. Her annual Case Managers Cruise is a fan favorite, where she gathers industry leaders to provide continuing education to case managers while sailing the Caribbean Sea.

Deanna has served on the Board of Directors of the CMSA Foundation, is a member of The Case Management Society of America (CMSA), Registered Nurse Innovators, Influencers, & Entrepreneurs (RNiie), The National Nurses In Business Association (NNBA), and Rotary where she currently sits on the board of directors for her local chapter. She is currently living her dream life in Puerto Aventuras, Mexico. From there she is writing her next book or course from her patio overlooking the beautiful Caribbean Sea.

Wendy Jaffe MSN RN CCM

Ms. Jaffe has been a staff nurse for 40 years, with the last 25 years as a certified case manager. She worked various staff and supervisory positions and went into case management when she landed a job at an insurance company. She worked there for three years and then transferred to a large city hospital. She was the stem cell/oncology case manager for 11 years, went to med/surg and then worked on the solid organ unit for the remainder of her time at this hospital. Ms. Jaffe retired from nursing on 1/25/2021! She states, "I will always be a nurse case manager and plan to do various nursing volunteer jobs. I am administering the COVID vaccines now and then we will see what lies ahead in my future?"

Jared 'Jay' Johnson MSW LMSW CCM

Jared Johnson "Jay" MSW LMSW CCM is the case management supervisor at Rehabilitation Hospital Navient Health inpatient rehabilitation facility in Macon Georgia. Jay's background includes working as a director of social services in a nursing home, an acute care case manager, and now his present role, as the case manager supervisor. Additionally, he serves as an adjunct as a local college in Macon Georgia teaching sophomore level social work courses. Jay was born and raised in west Texas. He received his Bachelor's in Social Work in San Angelo, Texas. He proceeded to pursue his Master's in Social Work in Arlington, Texas with a concentration in Children and Families. Jay is currently working towards his clinical licensure in social work.

Aishling Dalton Kelly CADDCT CFRDT CMDCP

A Public Speaker, toastmaster, and trainer. Aishling dedicates her life to seniors, their families, and caregivers advocating for all. Aishling presents an array of topics relative to home care. She has developed multiple programs on dementia for clients, caregivers, and health care professionals. She also holds multiple national certifications on Alzheimer's and dementia (CADDCT, CFRDT, CMDCP). She is a leader in the home care industry and has high standards for her caregivers and the families she encounters.

Anne Llewellyn RN-BC MS BHSA CCM CRRN

Anne Llewellyn is a nurse leader and passionate about the opportunities nurses have due to their education and expertise. Her goals are to empower and educate nurses in practice today, as well as those looking at nursing as a career option, to understand the opportunities nurses have in today's world of healthcare.

She has been a nurse for over 40 years, first as an LPN, and then as an RN. Her career has been "exciting and rewarding personally and professionally." She has worked in the hospital as a medical-surgical nurse, as a critical care nurse in the emergency department, and in the respiratory intensive care unit before moving into risk Management and then into case management and patient advocacy. She has been a business owner and also worked as an Editor in Chief for a National Healthcare Publication where she learned the power of the written word.

On November 24, 2014, Anne became a patient after being diagnosed with a brain tumor. This experience has renewed her energies as a nurse and an educator to work with patients and caregivers to help them better navigate the complex healthcare system. Today, Anne is a nurse advocate and a digital journalist, mentor and educator.

Mary Jo McHugh RN BSN

Mary Jo McHugh is a professional registered nurse with 30 years of experience in an urban, academic medical center with her last 20+ years dedicated to case management. Her experience as a case manager has ranged from entry level case management to being the manager of 18-21 professional nurse and social work team members with exceptional quality metrics including length of stay, patient satisfaction, and denial management. Mary Jo's strong clinical skills, leadership abilities, and recruitment efforts have developed, mentored, and trained nurse and social work professionals that have impacted patients' quality of life with positive outcomes.

Peter Miska RT

Pete Miska is a respiratory therapist and a thirty year veteran in the post acute care continuum. This includes the home health, home medical equipment, home infusion, and hospice industry. He has worked on multiple start ups of these types of companies and is a sought after speaker and advisor. Pete is an advocate of patient-centered care and the Triple Aim. He is also an active member of the CMSA , IHCC, COC, NASW and many other professional organizations. He can be reached at pmiska@aol.com.

Erika Peterson MSW LCSW

Erika Peterson MSW LCSW is a licensed clinical social worker who works at the University of Illinois at Chicago Hospital. She has twenty years of experience working with patients experiencing acute medical conditions and chronic mental health diagnoses. She has a passion working with patients from disadvantaged communities and linking patients with resources to overcome challenging social determinants of health. Erika has an emerging knowledge in trauma responsive treatments. In 2019, she received a CARE award after being recognized by the University of Illinois at Chicago Hospital for her commitment to her patients and strong advocacy work.

Metoda Posega RN CMSRN

Metoda Posega RN CMSRN and Certified Coder is the Senior Director of Business Development for Seasons Hospice and Palliative Care. Metoda has been a nurse for over 30 years and has experience in different nursing specialties. From working in the hospital setting on medical surgical units, to working in the emergency room, ICU, and post anesthesia care unit, to discharge planning, case management, and marketing for home health and hospice.

Hospice has been her passion for over 20 years. She worked in the hospice setting as a field case manager and also was a charge nurse for inpatient level of Hospice Care at MacNeal Hospital. Metoda conducted many in services on hospice care and discharge planning associated with end-of-life care at many area hospitals, nursing homes, and is still actively involved with teaching medical students and medical resident physicians. She is well known in the community for her knowledge of Hospice and end-of-life care.

Tonya O'Neill MSN RN CCM

Tonya O'Neil MSN RN CCM has dedicated her entire career of over 25 years as a registered nurse to working with the vulnerable, underserved, and most underrepresented members of our community. She worked as a community health nurse to expand health and wellness education within the faith community. She developed collaborative partnerships with grassroots organizations, local, and national organizations to create innovative ways to reach out to those in need.

She has held positions in home health as Director of Quality Assurance, overseeing quality improvement initiatives for home health, educating case managers on care coordination, and direct patient care. As a Patient Care Manager, she managed a large multidisciplinary team, her focus was excellent patient care, and care coordination that reduced unnecessary hospital readmissions.

She became certified as a Community Transitions Coach using the Eric Coleman Model with a large-scale collaborative Medicare project for county of San Diego, California. This award winning collaboration with multiple healthcare systems and the local agency on aging evolved into a replicable program that successfully reduced unnecessary readmissions through actively supporting patients to self-manage their health and coordinate their own care upon discharge from the acute care setting.

She then worked as a Regional Transitions Coordinator with a managed care Medicaid waiver program that offered an alternative to the dependance on nursing homes where individuals could safely return to their home with supportive community services. She volunteered within her community as an educator with the San Diego Black Nurses Association. Currently she is the Branch Director for Encompass Home Health and Hospice in Reston, Virginia. She is also an adjunct clinical professor of Community Health at Trinity Washington University in Washington, D.C. She earned a bachelor's degree in nursing and a master's degree in community health as an educator at Hampton University. She recently became a certified case manager who continues to promote health and wellness within her community.

Nancy Skinner RN BC CCM CMCN ACM-RN

Nancy Skinner has served as a case manager for the past 30 years, Director of Case Management, and an international case management educator. In her current role as principal consultant for Riverside HealthCare Consulting, she advances programs that promote excellence in care coordination and other transitional care strategies.

In 2002, she was named the Case Management Society of America (CMSA) National Case Manager of the Year and in 2008, she received CMSA's Lifetime Achievement Award. She currently serves as a Board Member for the Hospital Quality Foundation and as a reviewer for the Patient Centered Outcome Research Institute. Additionally, she assisted in the development of Post-Discharge Accreditation Standards for Cardiovascular Disease in partnership with the Society of Cardiovascular Patient Care.

Nancy is an Advisory Task Force Member of the National Transition of Care Coalition (NTOCC) as well as serving as Chair of NTOCC's Tools and Resources Committee. She is a member of both the Stakeholders Advisory Group for Project ACHIEVE and the Steering Committee for the Lambert Center for the Study of Medicinal Cannabis and Hemp. She is a Member of the Public Policy Committee for the American Case Management Society and a Member-At-Large for the Kentucky/Tennessee Chapter of the American Case Management Society. Nancy also served as primary faculty for the University of Southern Indiana Case Management Certificate Course for over 13 years.

Mariana Turgeon MSN RN CCM BSCS

Mariana Turgeon is a nurse case manager for a non-profit Catholic organization in Richmond, Virginia. After serving in the U.S. Navy, she pursued her Bachelor of Science in Computer Science (BSCS) at Strayer University in Woodbridge, Virginia, but knew the computer industry was not her passion. Mariana and her family decided this was the time for her to pursue her longtime desire of becoming a nurse and ultimately made the decision to enter nursing school in 1999, while working nights and raising two teenagers in Manassas, Virginia.

Fast forward, Mariana graduated in 2007 with her Associate's Degree in Nursing (ADN) from Northern Virginia Community College in Springfield, Virginia. While relocating to Powhatan County, Virginia (right outside the Richmond area), she worked as a labor and delivery nurse with the ultimate move into the pediatric ICU as a nurse case manager. She completed her BSN in 2014, and then her MSN in 2017 through the University of Phoenix. Just recently, she completed the Community Case Management (CCM) certification in August 2020.

Working with women and children has allowed her to care for the most vulnerable populations with the least resources. She continues to advocate for patients and families networking in the

Richmond community, as well as working as an adult care manager since the onset of COVID of 2020.

She has been married to Roger for 35 years. He works as an aircraft mechanic and they met in the Navy. Her daughter has followed her into labor and delivery nursing, graduating with her BSN in 2019, while raising her 14 year old son as a single mom. Her son just bought his first house after a stint in the U.S. Navy, currently evaluating diverse job opportunities for a longtime career.

Juliet B. Ugarte Hopkins MD CHCQM-PHYADV FABQAURP

Dr. Juliet Ugarte Hopkins is a graduate of the University of Illinois College of Medicine and served as co-chief resident while in her Pediatrics residency at Advocate Lutheran General Children's Hospital in Park Ridge, Illinois. Dr. Ugarte Hopkins practiced as a pediatric hospitalist for a decade and also served as medical director of pediatric hospital medicine and vice-chair of pediatrics at Rockford Health System in Rockford, Illinois before transitioning into her current role as the first Physician Advisor for Case Management, Utilization, and Clinical Documentation at ProHealth Care, Inc., a two-hospital, 575-bed health system in Southeastern Wisconsin.

Dr. Ugarte Hopkins is board-certified in health care quality and management with a physician advisor sub-specialty by the American Board of Quality Assurance and Utilization Physicians (ABQAURP). She is the first physician board member for the Wisconsin chapter of the American Case Management Association (ACMA), a member of the RAC Monitor editorial board, and she was recognized as a "Hirsch's Hero" by Dr. Ronald Hirsch in 2016.

She lives with her husband in northern Illinois where they valiantly strive to raise three daughters and a son into strong, thoughtful, and self-assured individuals with a corny sense of humor.

Ellen Walker LCSW ACSW

Ellen Parucka Walker LCSW ACSW Received her Bachelor of Social Work at George Williams College in Downers Grove, Illinois and her Master of Social Work at Jane Addams College of Social Work, University of Illinois at Chicago. For the past three years she has been the social work manager at West Suburban Medical Center in Oak Park, Illinois and has worked there as a social worker for the past 26 years. She also has experience working as a senior services case worker at what is now working at Aging Care Connections in La Grange, Illinois. Her past experience includes working as a crisis worker for a teenage crisis agency and her internship at Hines VA Hospital. She is a member of the National Association of Social Workers and the Case Managers Society of America.

Charles White EdD MBA CPHQ

Dr. White has over 25 years of healthcare leadership, governance, and systems improvement experience. He holds a Bachelor's degree in Hospital Administration and Planning from the University of New Hampshire, a Master's degree in Business Administration and Planning from Southern University of New Hampshire, and a Doctorate in Education from Capella University. Dr. White has a passion for engaging stakeholders in innovative change, operational results, and hardwiring system change to improve the delivery of patient care to vulnerable and at-risk populations. He is faculty in the Department of Public Health at California State University Fullerton.

Anna Rheka Winkowski MSN RN CCM ACM-RN

Anna is a graduate of Aurora University and has a Bachelor of Science in Nursing. Anna has dual masters, first in Health Services Administration from National Louis University, and second in Medical Informatics from Northwestern University. She is a certified case manager (CCM) and an accredited case manager (ACM). She is an active member with the Case Management Society of America and American Case Management Association. Anna has a green belt in Lean Six Sigma.

As a Health Network Strategy Executive at Cerner Corporation, Anna works with executive and senior clinical, business and technical leadership to ensure alignment of population health solutions and strategies with overall objectives to obtain expected results and value. She makes an impact on Cerner/clients by helping them establish care management goals, strategies and objectives that support population health management and the transition to emerging payment models.

ABOUT THE AUTHOR

Colleen Morley DNP RN CCM CMAC CMCN ACM-RN, is the Regional Director of Case Management for Pipeline Health, overseeing case management operations in Illinois facilities. Prior to this role, Dr. Morley has held positions of leadership in acute care settings as the Director of Case Management to oversee utilization review, case management, and social services at several Chicago area hospitals. She has also held leadership positions at managed care organizations as the Director of Case Management and Manager of Health Services. She has focused on piloting quality improvement initiatives that emphasized readmission reduction and improved care coordination through effective communication, and population health management for acute care, managed care and community care settings. Through these initiatives, she has been an "advocate for the advocates" by supporting the case management community.

Dr. Morley has over 20 years of nursing experience. Her clinical nursing specialties include medical/surgical, oncology, and pediatrics. She received her Associate's Degree in Nursing (ADN) at South Suburban College in South Holland, Illinois. She earned her Bachelor's of Science in Nursing degree (BSN) at Jacksonville University in Jacksonville, Florida and her Master's of Science in Nursing (MSN) from Norwich University in Northfield, Vermont. At Chamberlain College of Nursing, she achieved her Doctorate in Nursing Practice (DNP).

She currently serves in many roles:

President Elect; CMSA National Board of Directors (2021-2022)

Past President; CMSA Chicago (2021-2023)

Vice President; CMSA Foundation (2021-2022)

Secretary/PAC Treasurer/Trustee/ Legislative Chair; ANA-Illinois (2019-2021)

Acting Secretary/Director; Illinois Nurses' Foundation Board

Member of Advisory Board; Case Management Monthly

Member of Editorial Board; Professional Case Management Journal

Member; National Associate of Healthcare Revenue Improvement Leadership Council

In 2010, Dr. Morley received the Managed Care Nurse Leader of the Year award from AAMCN for her work in updating the CMCN curriculum and study program. In 2020, she was the recipient of the CMSA Foundation Practice Improvement Award and the ANA Illinois Clinical Improvement Award for her work on the important topic of health literacy promotion.

She is the proud mother of three incredible adult children (Caitlyn, Connor, and Cristian), grandmother of one (Bram Connor), and pack leader for a herd of chihuahua friends (Carina, Marilyn, and Yoda). Her hobbies include reading, quilting, watching movies, enjoying live music, traveling, and watching documentaries on true crime, history, and art history.